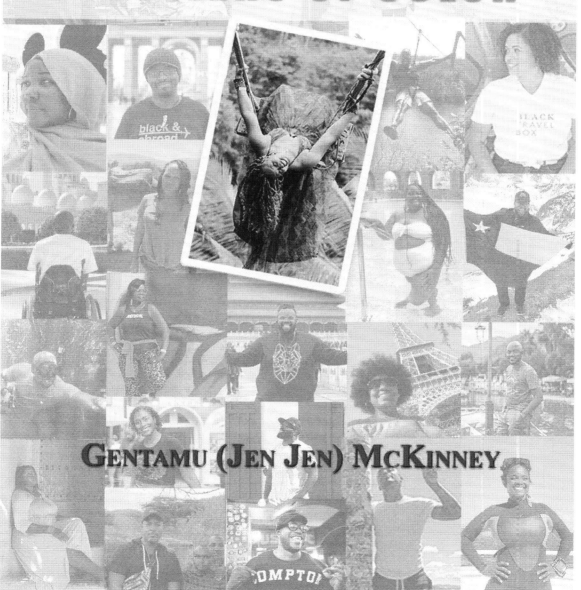

Keep Calm, Bring Your Carry On!
THE ULTIMATE SELFCARE GUIDE FOR
TRAVELERS OF COLOR

GENTAMU (JEN JEN) MCKINNEY

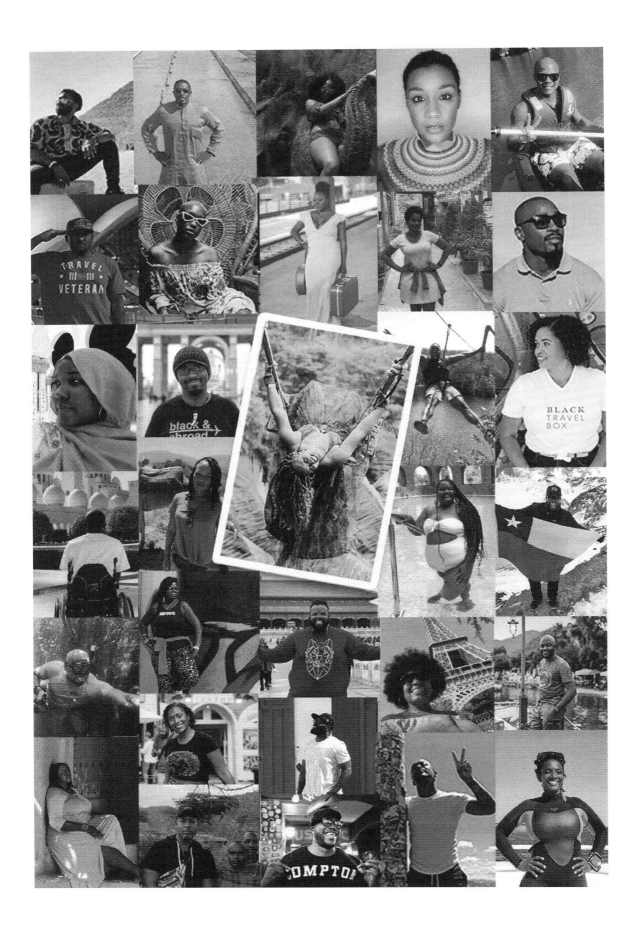

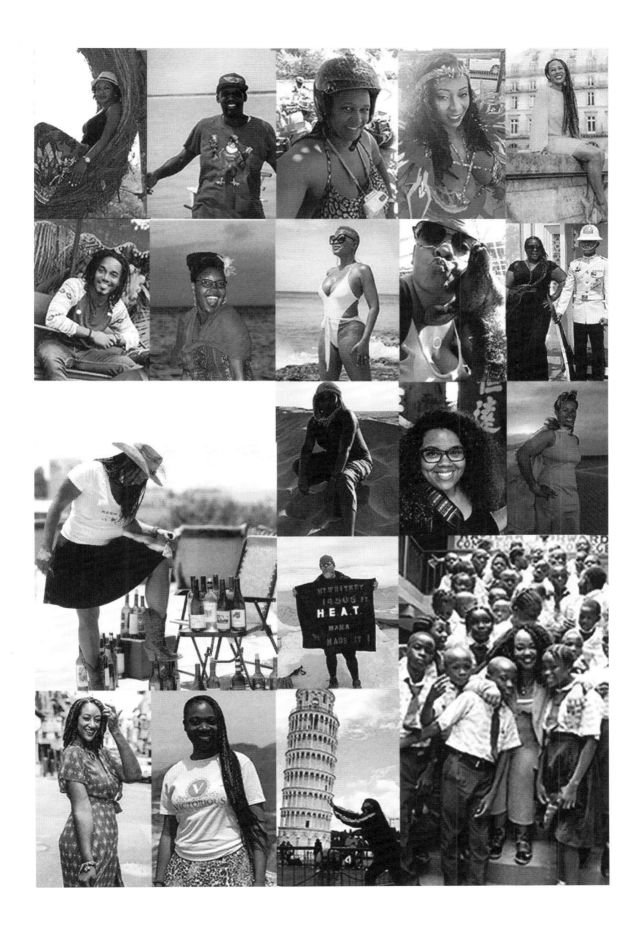

Copyright © 2020 by Gentamu (Jen Jen) McKinney

All rights reserved. This book or any portion thereof may not be reproduced or used in any manner whatsoever without the express written permission of the publisher except for the use of brief quotations in a book review.

Printed in the United States of America

First Printing, 2020

ISBN:

TABLE OF CONTENTS

Chapter 1: Gentamu (Jen Jen) McKinney...1

Chapter 2: Evita Robinson 9

Chapter 3: Fletcher Cleaves 15

Chapter 4: Jeff Jenkins 20

Chapter 5: Jerry C' Way 25

Chapter 6: Dana Armstead 31

Chapter 7: Omoruyi Osagiede 37

Chapter 8: Ejide Fashina 43

Chapter 9: Paul Bashea Williams 49

Chapter 10: Marilene Shane 54

Chapter 11: Kurtis Henry 60

Chapter 11 Continued: Jakarri Stroman 66

Chapter 12: Tomiko Harvey 72

Chapter 13: Brian Oliver 78

Chapter 14: La Tessa Montgomery 83

Chapter 15: Akeem Tolson 90

Chapter 16: Nubia Young..95

Chapter 17: Gabbok..100

Chapter 18: Nicole Brewer 105

Chapter 19: Darnell Walker 109

Chapter 20: Sonjia Mackey 114

Chapter 21: Leroy Tyler 120

Chapter 22: Eartha Franklin 125

Chapter 23: Stan Miles 131

Chapter 24: Jill Carter 136

Chapter 25: Roland Parker...141

Chapter 26: Slyvia (Sly) Callendar 146

Chapter 27: Fanon Wilkins 153

Chapter 28: Mahogany Ratcliffe 158

Chapter 29: Brett Roberts..163

Chapter 30: Stephanie Snipes 168

Chapter 31: Yahya Bey 174

Chapter 32: Kristen Riddle 179

Chapter 33: Dr. Keyon Anderson 185

Chapter 34: Shani Brinkley 190

Chapter 35: Michael Agyin 195

Chapter 36: Tuanni Price 201

Chapter 37: Nicole Vick 206

Chapter 38: Orion Brown 211

Chapter 39: Martinique Lewis 217

Chapter 40: Tammy Freeman 222

Chapter 41: Kristin Riddle 228

Chapter 42: Karlyn Le Blanc 234

Chapter 43: Tiffany Heard 239

Chapter 44: Shanayla Sweat 244

Chapter 45: Adrienne Ferguson 249

Chapter 46: Tiffany Wright 255

Chapter 47: Nykki Allen 260

Chapter 48: Yvette Christopher 265

Chapter 49: Lorena Garduno 271

Chapter 50: Frances Armad 276

Chapter 51: Roshida Dowe 281

Chapter 52: Javonne Sanders 285

Chapter 53: Hooda Brown 290

Mental Health Awareness Observances & Resources and Apps.............................297

DEDICATION

To my grandmother: you are my heart. Words can't express the amount of gratitude I have for the amount of love and wisdom you poured into me. Although I could never take my mother's place, I hope the love I have shown you throughout the years has filled the void of not having her fully in your life. I know your time here will end soon. Don't worry about me for you have fully prepared me for your departure. All I ask is that you just check on me from time to time so I can feel your presence. Thank you for giving me some of the best experiences a granddaughter could ever have

To my mother: your mental health diagnosis and experience that we shared getting you through was not in vain. You have aligned me with my purpose to help release others from their mental prison.

To my Dad: Thanks for laying the Foundation The "Mckinney" Legacy of giving back to our community continues.

Chasity Signers Dr. Connie Mitchell. Juanita Williams, Jayla Braxtar, Nicole Vick, Cacy Duncan, Ann Charles: Thank you for helping me through this. Its been one helluva emotional rollercoaster

To my adoptive Mothers Rhonda Bean and Denise Gordan: Thanks for loving me like your own

To Rhonda Dennis: Thanks for being that that older sibling that I never got to experience as a child

To my travel colleagues,Travel Hero's and She-ro's :Thank you for trusting me with your stories and coming together as one to fight something bigger than ourselves

I really didn't understand it at first but I want to thank God for using me as a vessel to gather all these handpicked individuals to address something that is not only dear to my heart but is also a worldwide issue

Cover Art design and concept by Gentamu McKinney
Art Illustration by John Barge III

MY WHY

Several years ago, out of nowhere my mother had a mental health breakdown. This was shocking to me because according to studies my mother had characteristics of an Alpha female. I am here to say they are all wrong. I have never seen her like that before. One minute she was angry and within 5 minutes she had shown me several different personalities. She had even contemplated suicide. I remember thinking she probably just relapsed from being 14 years clean and sober. After repeated test lab test from the emergency room, there were no signs of drugs or physical head trauma. From there her world and mine were turned completely upside down financially, spiritually, mentally and physically. It would also lead to my life long journey of mental health advocacy in the African American communities.

As the years went by, I had several minority mental health events within my community, sold mental health awareness apparel and office swag, directed and produced a "Let's Get Mental; a documentary about mental health awareness and stigma behind it in the African American communities, art and play therapy with children abroad in improvise communities. In 2019, I was even one of the recipients of the 40 under 40 award for my mental health advocacy in the African American communities but I still felt like I wasn't doing enough. Through my travels, I saw that mental health awareness was needed on a worldwide scale. I wanted to do more and have more a global impact. Now how was little ol me going to do that? The vision was very clear but looking for the steps or instructions to get there was very foggy at the time and then it just came to me.

The sudden death of Anthony Bourdain had shocked the travel world to its core. The industry could no longer ignore the correlation between travel and mental health. Within the past 2 years, there has been an influx of people not just going on vacations but trying to find healing and a deeper connection with the world and themselves. This includes mind,body and spiritual retreats, adult gap years, solo travel and voluntourism also known as give-cations or travelanthropy.

Some have asked, "Why would you limit your audience to just people of color and travelers? that doesn't make sense." These questions got me feeling like ol boy from the movie "Love Jones ". So let me break this shit down for you so it can be forever and consistently be broken.

1) "Why the F#$%@ not? Our ancestors were kidnapped, placed on slave ships, and sold into slavery all across the world. As far as I'm concern, that's where the generational mental health trauma began. I'm not limiting myself at all. I am making an impact by providing awareness, education, and healing by revisiting where we started from.

2) In the climate that we live in today, Being black is lit but is its also stressful than a mutha f!@#$ and it can get you killed. It comes with generations of trauma. My book coach said no cursing but I'll be damn if I censor myself in my own damn book, I get enough of that shit at work! In my NeNe Voice, "I said, What I said.

My Why

3) Black doesn't crack physically, however we are dying on the inside. Most of us suffer in silence because talking about it or going to see a counselor or therapist is viewed as weak or crazy Suicide rates amongst African Americans have doubled over the past several years.

4) Cabin fever is real! The need to just get out,leave it all behind and just carry all your essentials and favorite items in one bag and buy shit when you get there.

So what is the objective of this book ? To give you some practical baby steps towards obtaining optimal mental health when in route to your next destination, while at home or at work. Will this book solve all your problems Hell to No ! This book will not solve all your mental health problems nor was it meant to during its creation. We highly encourage you to seek professional help,support groups and other mental health support tools! However, this book will for damn sure help you realize that you are not alone and you do not have to suffer in silence.

It will educate, empower encourage you to take more care of your mental health just as your physical all while exploring different parts of the world.

Without further due Welcome to Let's Get Mental Airlines a subsidy of Work n Play Co. Flight 2020 departing LAX to optimal mental wellness. My name is Gentamu (Jen Jen) McKinney, I am your captain and this is my flight crew. We are going to take you on a beautiful journey. So Keep Calm and Bring your Carry on!

Over 50 passports

Over 500 Passport stamps

Over 1 million sky miles

One Goal:
Breaking the silence and stigma about mental health in
black communities worldwide

CHAPTER 1

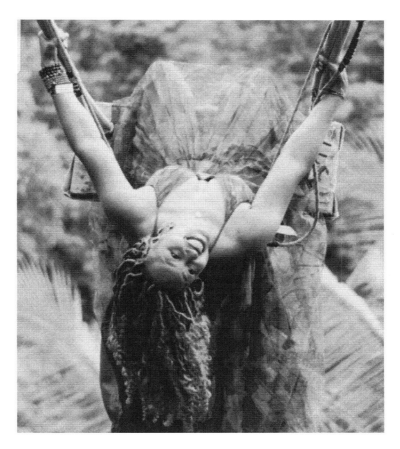

Gentamu (Jen Jen) McKinney

The Advocate
Sometimes I work, Sometimes I play,
and Sometimes I do both

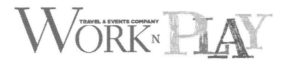

Where Adventure & Social Responsibility Collide

Travel Quote or Travel Mantra you live by
Don't Just See the World, Give Back to it

Travel Influencer/ Brand Summary

Work N Play is an adventure and social responsibility company. We combine volunteerism, therapeutic play and wellness with events and travel excursions. Our areas of focus are Corporate events, Employee wellness, Teambuilding, Therapeutic play for adults, Travel Health and Volunteer cultural exchanges abroad formally known as voluntourism. We help create the perfect work and play environment.

How has Traveling helped you maintain your mental health as it relates to self-care?

Traveling is part of my self-care routine rather it be local or international. I like to call it to travel therapy. It allows me to recharge and heal myself mentally, physically and spiritually. It also allows me to silent in my thoughts and places things and situations in its proper perspective. It has helped me appreciate the more simpler things in life and made feel more comfortable in my own skin. Traveling the world and giving back while doing it has brought a sense of calmness to my life.

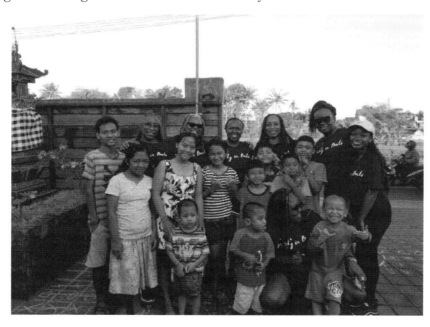

Gentamu (Jen Jen) McKinney

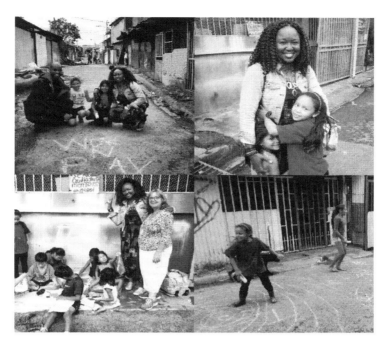

What is your most therapeutic travel destination for stress relief and self-care?

Hands down Bali! It is one of the enchanting and spiritual places that I have ever been to. I like to call it my second home this is my go-to place for ultimate mental, physical and spiritual healing. As soon as you touch the ground you immediately feel the weight of the world lifted off your shoulders. I felt like I could breathe again.

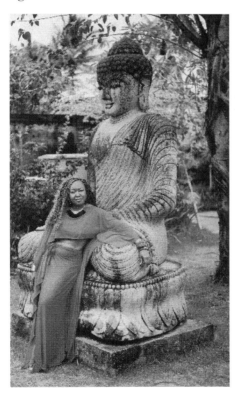
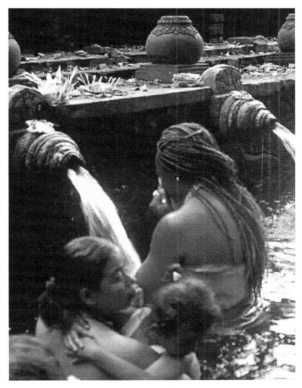

Whats is the most important items you have in your carryon and why?

1) As a certified germaphobe who works for in healthcare and teaches infection control for a living, disinfectant wipes and hand sanitizer are first on my list with the song " Wipe Me Down" by Webbie playing in the background **2)** My Epi-pen because my life depends on it! I usually bring 2 to 3 depending on the length of the trip **3)** Dental Hygiene products because fresh travel breath is important. you never know who you may meet wink wink. Right now I am loving Listerene's new mouthwash tablets **3)** Extra set of underwear and body hygiene products such as a honey pot. After an airline lost my luggage I vowed to never get caught slipping again **4)** Florida water – immediately rids bad Juju and protects your energy. Its light fragrance gives helps with its calming travel anxiety **5)** My healing crystals **6)** My mini singing bowl **7)** mini sage **8)**prayer beads. Mini-Mental health affirmation candles by Light the Mood Candle Company and Concrete Rose. **9)** My USB Travel aroma diffuser **10)** Traveler's cocktail kits The old fashion and Moscow Mule are my favorite **11)** Flex Menstrual cup and honest Organic Pads for when Aunt Flo wants to have her own unsolicited vacation and itinerary. **12)** My Surface Pro by Microsoft because work comes first then I play **13)** Rose Gold Beats by Dre **15)** Smucker's Uncrustables because peanut butter and jelly are my favorite and its packaged well for flights **16)** My Pocket Moleskine because I was told it was for writers and I was like well.... I am a writer damn it !

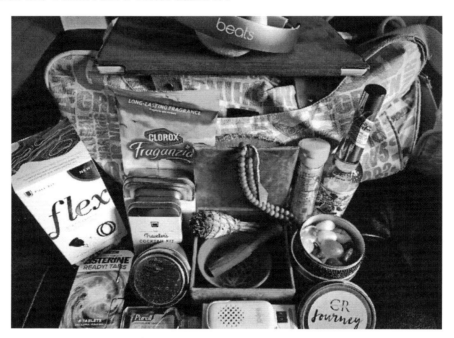

Favorite Calming Beverage or Food to consume while traveling and why?

I am either drinking wine, some type of alcoholic cocktail or calming tea. My go-to is the " Carry on cocktail kit " Old fashion and Moscow Mule. its a kit that includes everything you need to make your favorite cocktails mid-flight.its also TSA approved

Favorite Keepsake that keeps you calm or grounded while traveling?

My heart My granny

Gentamu (Jen Jen) McKinney

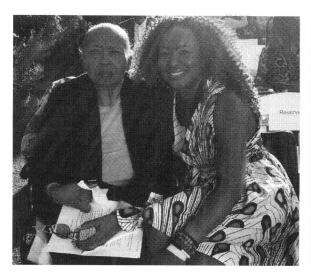
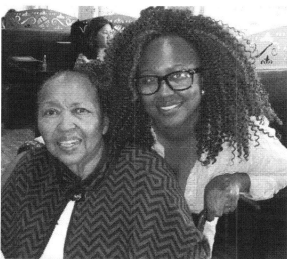

What is your most hilarious travel memory?

I Work N Plays group trip to Bangkok and Phuket. The whole trip was pure F$#@* -ing comedy From start to finish comedy. Nonstop laughter.

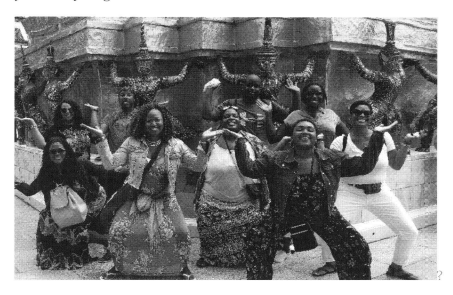

What is your most memorable or touching travel experience?

Work This would have been a tie between our trip to Costa Rica and Bali. Each trip involves a volunteer project. In Bali and Costa Rica, we did therapeutic play and art therapy with kids who were less fortunate. We also donated hygiene supplies and clothes. However in Bali, I decided to do something a little different since I had an all women's group for the first time. Not gonna lie I was a little nervous but I felt like God was telling me that these groups needed something different. After having several conversations with each of the guests, I decided to add a mental health component for them. With the help of my colleague Hasna from More than Just Drums Healing Vibrations, I was able to add vibrational sound healing and a sister circle component. I never really knew how much it was needed until the ladies filled the room with heartbreak, decades of generational trauma and a waterfall of tears. It was an instant purge and they had been released from whatever was keeping them hostage from living freely and peacefully.

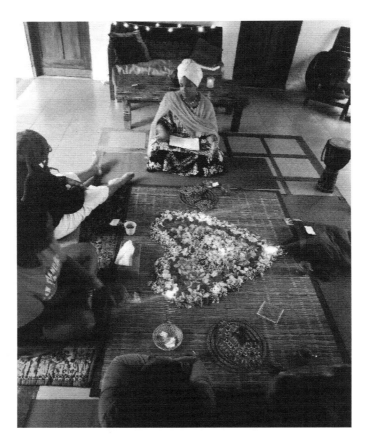

What is the worst travel experience you ever had?

As a trip coordinator you always try to plan for the unexpected, but the truth of the matter is Shit Happens. It's a part of this thing called life. It doesn't smell good or look good and nobody wants to touch it. However, it has its place and its all in how you handle it so that it is properly contained. Just pray there is always toilet paper around to clean up the mess, a universal toilet instead of a squat and understanding and flexible group trip mates. Giving your guest a heads up is always helpful too. In the words of the late John Witherspoon " Don't nobody go into the bathroom for about 35- 45 minutes."

Favorite Travel Hack?

If you forgot to purchase a foldable bag, grab a plastic or reusable grocery bag to rid of extra items that may cause your luggage to be overweight.

Activated charcoal is Travel Bible don't @ me !

What is your travel Ritual for keeping calm and maintaining your inner zen?

I have travel candles especially designed for my needs by Light the mood. Every morning I pray, meditate and repeat positive affirmations from You are Creators (a popular meditation youtube channel) while burning sage, or playing my singing bowl or my sound healing app. I also keep healing stones around me that are specific to my needs. I also take the time to be completely by myself with mother nature listening to the sounds of the earth and taking it all in

Why is addressing mental health and self-care as it relates to people of color so important in the travel community?

The truth of the matter is Black doesn't crack on the outside but on the inside it hurts like hell. We are dying at an alarming rate mentally from years of generational trauma and unconsciously using travel as a method of therapy but still ashamed to come forth that mentally we are not healthy and get the proper tools to deal with it due to the stigma. Black people are taught to work hard because due to an unfair system we had to. However we were never taught self-care as it relates to mental health only physical.

Although we travel often for our mental health, the topic is not emphasized due to shame and stigma. How can we normalize this conversation among the travel communities of color?

This can be done by curating nontraditional and unconventional platforms like this book where the masses can see and hear from people that not only look like them but provide tools and resources. Each year not just talk about mental health but also provide. For example each year I put on a mental health event called "Let's Get Mental for Minority Mental Health Awareness month along with selling trendy mental health awareness apparel and office swag. I also had the opportunity to host this year's Millennial Mental Health Expo put on by the City of Los Angele's Empowerment Congress and speak at this year's Audacity festivals Mental Health & Travel Panel.

WEBSITE

www.worknplayco.com

EMAIL

info@worknplayco.com

worknplaytravel@gmail.com

awarenessafterdark@gmail.com

INSTAGRAM HANDLE

https://www.instagram.com/worknplayco

https://www.instagram.com/voluntouradventures

https://www.instagram.com/awarenessafterdark

FACEBOOK PAGE

https://www.facebook.com/worknplaytravel

https://www.facebook.com/awarenessafterdark

Travel Jokes

"You travel too much."

ME: ✈️✈️✈️✈️ ✈️

CHAPTER 2

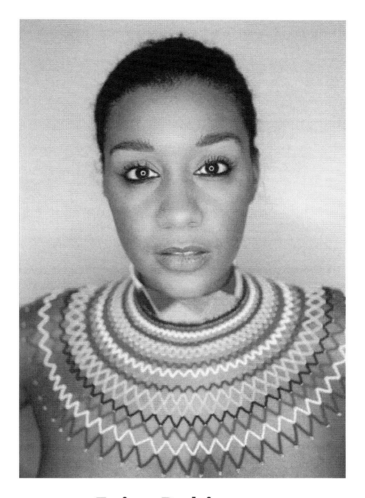

Evita Robinson

The God Mother of Travel

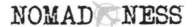

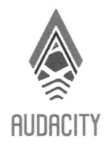

Travel Quote or Travel Mantra you live by
Don't get Hung up on the Fear of Travel.... Just Start

Travel Influencer/ Brand Summary

Nomadness Travel Tribe is an online social travel community that primarily targets Black and Brown millennials. Audacity Fest was birthed due to the huge success of Nomadness Tribe. Audacity Fest is a festival that celebrates and creates a safe place for travelers of color to discuss issues centered around them.

How has Traveling helped you maintain your mental health as it relates to self-care?

Travel for me is about the escape. Although it can be seen as a form of escapism however. There is a warrior in me that comes alive and not being held down by physical and emotional luggage. Where ever I go there is an energy change

What is your most therapeutic travel destination for stress relief and self-care?

For a dose of humility, I go to India. This is a different type of self-care for me because it always puts things in perspective. When I leave I don't leave complaining, I am more appreciative of the things that I have and able to do. One of the things I love about India is the festival of Colors. In Turkey they do the call of prayer. Although I am not Islamic hearing it is very meditative and its something that resonates with me and gives me a sense of stress relief. This but being a creative writers retreat for me It is a very majestic place.

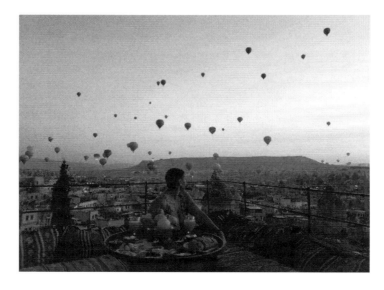

Evita Robinson

What's is the most important items you have in your carryon and why?
> My cell phone, charger, journal, headphones and laptop

Favorite Calming Beverage or Food to consume while traveling and why?
> Any type of green tea

Favorite Calming Music or Audio to listen to while traveling?
> I am a big fan of Jhnike Aniko. Her new sound bath Trigger Warnings Mantras are the shit ! she just has such an amazing angelic voice. Also Guided meditations by Tara Brock. My therapist recommended her its like a tranquilizer they knock me out Soundbaths Sound baths

Favorite Keepsake that keeps you calm or grounded while traveling?
> Journals would definitely be my number one. I have to be able to write and get my thoughts out I even buy journals abroad. If I see one that I really like that I feel like I cant get at home, I will buy it an start writing in it when I get home.

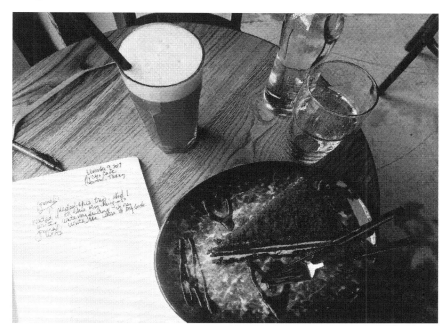

What is your most memorable or touching travel experience?
> Before I die Wall in Johannesburg. You can read people's inserts and look into people's lives on what they want to do before they die.

What is the worst travel experience you ever had?
> All of my trips have been full of blessings and a lot of lessons. Sometimes there were certain things that were just out of my control and you gotta face the music head-on and take responsibility. However, as long as I show up I know the warrior in me will come out and figure it out. I don't just show up when it's pretty for awards, magazine covers and accolades, I show up when it's pretty shitty too!

Favorite Travel Hack?
> oregano and compression socks. Oregano is the cure for everything I swear!

What is your travel Ritual for keeping calm and maintaining your inner zen?

Chakra clearings and Reiki. Right now I've been really into kickboxing

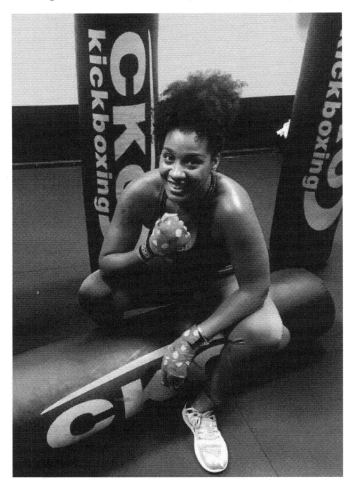

Best Travel Tip Advice?

Find Your tribe

Why is addressing mental health in and self-care with as it relates to people of color so important in the travel community?

When it comes to mental health as it relates to people of color, we have unique experiences and traumas. We have unique experiences and trauma. And unique systems that. Travel is our lives' current manifestation of breaking through all that. We owe it to the next generation to do the healing necessary to break the cycle

Although we travel often for our mental health, the topic is not emphasized due to shame and stigma. How can we normalize this conversation among the travel communities of color?

I have always been a mental health advocate. I've been seeing a therapist probably since I was about 12 or 13 years old. I even share my own personal struggles and journey with anxiety via my Facebook lives. I believe that creating spaces where others can speak freely without judgment can change the narrative. I would get so much engagement when I did address mental health via social media, I decided to add a mental health & travel component to this year's Audacity Festival.

Evita Robinson

WEBSITE

https://www.nomadnesstv.com/

https://www.audacityfest.com

https://www.evitarobinson.com/

EMAIL

info@audacityfest.com

Info@nomadnesstv.com

INSTAGRAM HANDLE

Audacityfest

Nomadness Tribe

FACEBOOK PAGE

Audacityfest

Nomadness Tribe

Travel Jokes

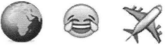

I asked HR for leave and they declined. I appealed HR's response and it's now sitting on the Managing Director's desk. Managing Director is me, I am the Managing Director, the Managing Director is I.

CHAPTER 3

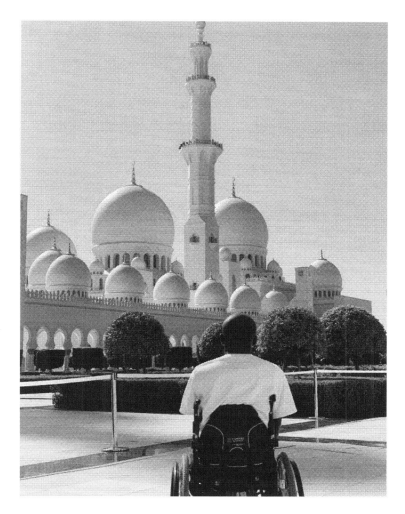

Fletcher Cleaves
Picture me Rollin

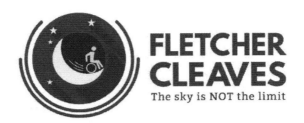

Travel Quote or Travel Mantra you live by
This Wheelchair won't stop me! The Sky is NOT the Limit

Travel Influencer/ Brand Summary

The Sky is NOT the Limit is a slogan adopted by Fletcher Cleaves. How can we say the sky is the limit when there are footprints on the moon! Fletcher encourages people to live life to the fullest no matter your current circumstances! Travel and explore the world! Life is meant to be lived! Life is not about what happens to you! Bad stuff happens to everybody! It's how you respond to adversity and when things don't go your way that defines who you are!

How has Traveling helped you maintain your mental health as it relates to self-care?

When my car accident happened in 2009 that left me paralyzed and losing my football scholarship I was depressed because I couldn't play anymore. But once I discovered a love for traveling things began to change drastically. Traveling is the one thing that makes me feel free and without a disability. With every new city, with every new country... I feel a little less disabled as if I can conquer the world!

What is your most therapeutic travel destination for stress relief and self-care?

It varies! Sometimes I may need to go to a beach in the Caribbean and clear my mind. Sometimes I may feel adventurous and eat fresh escargot in Paris. Or sometimes I may feel like a thrill seeker and ride the world's fastest rollercoaster in Abu Dhabi

What's is the most important items you have in your carryon and why?

My situation is a little different. The most important items I have are my medical supplies

Favorite Calming Beverage or Food to consume while traveling and why?

I honestly don't have one. I typically go around the world tasting various Long Island's hahaha. Something about a Long Island Ice Tea that loosens me up lol

Favorite Calming Music or Audio to listen to while traveling?

Music is Life! It helps me on long flights, loosen up, etc. I listen to Hip Hop, Blues, R&B, Soul, almost anything lol

Favorite Keepsake that keeps you calm or grounded while traveling?

I just pray and get on my way.

What is your most hilarious travel memory?

My brother and I were trying to take a silly picture in front of the Eiffel Tower and this random keep creeping into our pics lol

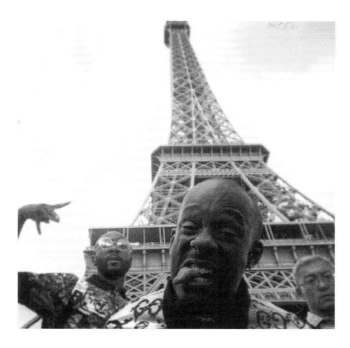

What is your most memorable or touching travel experience?

>All my vacations are memorable. I treat each as if it were my last.

What is the worst travel experience you ever had?

>Flying from Rome to Paris, the airline lost my wheelchair and I had to just wait on the plane for an hour and a half

Favorite Travel Hack?

>N/A

What is your travel Ritual for keeping calm and maintaining your inner zen?

>Listen to Music

Best Travel Tip Advice?

>Don't stress. Enjoy the vacation.

Why is addressing mental health in and self-care with as it relates to people of color so important in the travel community?

>As a Black man we typically are taught to not show emotion, be tough, etc. Traveling can help express feelings and emotions. Seeing one of the 7 wonders of the world could help them feel inner peace or new emotions.

Although we travel often for our mental health, the topic is not emphasized due to shame and stigma. How can we normalize this conversation among the travel communities of color?

>Not being ashamed comes from within. You have to feel comfortable enough within to not be ashamed of things that help your mental health

The Ultimate Self-Care Guide for Travelers of Color

WEBSITE

www.fletchercleaves.com

EMAIL

fletchercleaves@gmail.com

INSTAGRAM HANDLE

@RollinOnFaith

FACEBOOK PAGE

@Fletcher Cleaves

Travel Jokes

I identify as a carry on bag. You will now let me fly anywhere for $30.

> **United Airlines** ✓ @united
> Fly how you identify. Our new non-binary gender options are now available.

CHAPTER 4

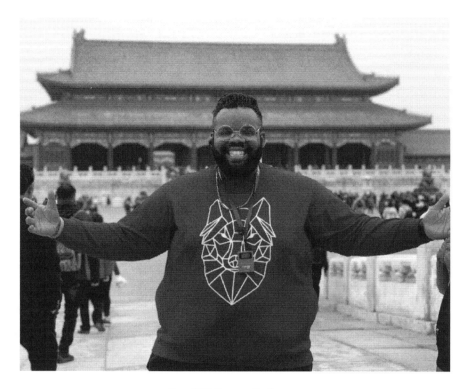

Jeff Jenkins
Chubby Diaries

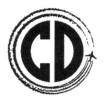

Travel Quote or Travel Mantra you live by
Live Life Now

Travel Influencer / Brand Summary
We help Chubby People travel around the world!

How has Traveling helped you maintain your mental health as it relates to self-care?
Traveling has helped my mental health in a few ways. 1. The long plane rides or hanging out in nature give me ample opportunity for introspection. I get to refocus on my personal why, dream without distractions, and reflect on what there is to be grateful for. 2. Travel gives me the option to learn things I didn't know, connect with people I never met, and all of these experiences have helped me disrupt bias I once had. Which helps me be a better global citizen and an overall better me.

What is your most therapeutic travel destination for stress relief and self-care?
Belize has been by far one of my most reflective and stress relieving destination! I got to literally sit in the ocean with drinks for hours. Belize is so laid back, stress-free atmosphere and you get the whole tropical vibes. It brought relaxation and inspiration the entire time I was there

What's is the most important items you have in your carryon and why?
My MacBook Pro! I read books off my Mac, watch movies, download videos from my camera so that I can edit them later. Since I travel for a living having my MacBook I'm about to do work from anywhere

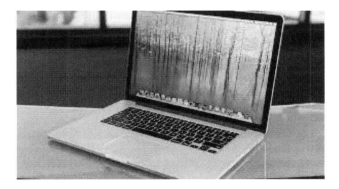

Favorite Calming Beverage or Food to consume while traveling and why?
I love margaritas. Seriously, I equate Margaritas to being on vacation or it's time to relax mode. I love the citrus taste and tequila also lowers your blood pressure so you feel more relaxed

Favorite Calming Music or Audio to listen to while traveling?
I listen to Baby bedtime sounds and one I listen to off that album is Oceans. So it is a constant white noise vibe

Favorite Keepsake that keeps you calm or grounded while traveling? (ex. Pic of loved one, jewelry, gifted item)

My backpack! I take it everywhere with me, and it def keeps me grounded and means so much to me.

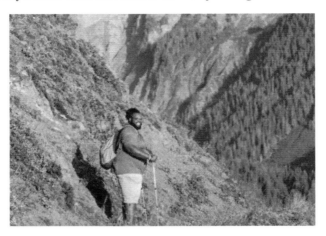

What is your most hilarious travel memory?

I believe I was in Thailand and a group of travelers and I were walking for some reason 4 of us all tripped over this uneven pavement and that became the joke of the weekend. It actually brought us all together

What is your most memorable or touching travel experience?

My most memorable travel experience was traveling for the first time to another country and that country was Japan. Being inundated by a new culture, new foods, and traditions I was so taken back and in awe. It made such an impacted on me that 15 years later I still am traveling around the world

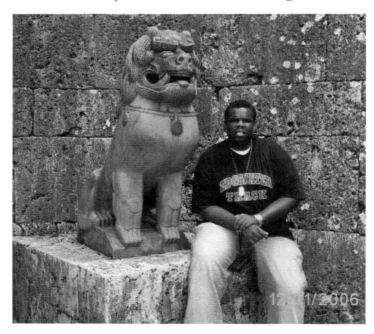

What is the worst travel experience you ever had?

Being in Thailand. I am not going to say I didn't enjoy myself but if I didn't go back there again I would be ok. I thought it was over touristic and didn't enjoy all that I saw there. And on top of that my leg feel through the floor of a deck and I bruised myself very badly

Jeff Jenkins

Favorite Travel Hack?

Not buying my hotel until the day before. I literally have saved so much money doing it!

What is your travel Ritual for keeping calm and maintaining your inner Zen?

Staying grateful and having no expectations. If I continue to be and do these two then I will have an incredible time and people around me will as well!

Best Travel Tip Advice?

I want to speak to my plus-size community. I know that our weight can get in our way but we don't have to let that stop us from living our best lives now!

Why is addressing mental health in and self-care with as it relates to people of color so important in the travel community?

Addressing mental in the POC travel space is so important because traditionally we haven't been able to condition not to seek out help or give our minds and bodies the proper self-care it needs and deserves.

Although we travel often for our mental health, the topic is not emphasized due to shame and stigma. How can we normalize this conversation among the travel communities of color??

I first think it is powerful to give POCs permission to actually go. I have empowered so many people to seek help and told them it is ok that they did because not only worsens the situation. Also if I model it people are more likely to think that if Jeff went and it was a benefit to him then I should as well

WEBSITE

Chubbydiaries.com

EMAIL

jeff@chubbydiaries.com

INSTAGRAM HANDLE

@chubbydiaries__

Travel Jokes

  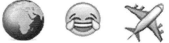

My wife is amazing. For my b-day she purchased a $250k life insurance policy and a trip to the Dominican Republic. 😄😄

CHAPTER 5

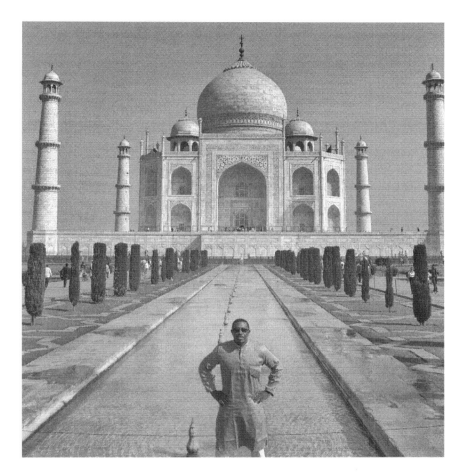

Jerry C' Way

Travel FreQk

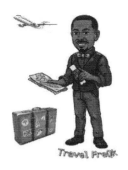

Travel Quote or Travel Mantra you live by
When we leaving?

Travel Influencer/ Brand Summary

I Live For A Living

How has Traveling helped you maintain your mental health as it relates to self-care??

I've battled depression stemming from my accident back in 2015. So when I say travel is my therapy, I really mean it. While travel isn't a panacea against depression and mental health, it has definitely given me coping skills. Travel for me creates inspiration which can help alter one's perceptions of ourselves and those around us. Sometimes depression causes you to have an outlook on life that involves a skewed view of the world. However, traveling allows me to literally see the bigger picture. It can help me put certain thoughts and beliefs into perspective in a way I think more candidly. When we remove ourselves out of our usual environment, we are forced to literally see the world from a different perspective.

What is your most therapeutic travel destination for stress relief and self-care?

My favorite destination for stress relief and self-care would be Diani Beach in Kenya which is right outside of Mombasa. The white sand is so soft and feels as if you're walking on silk. Crystal clear water and you can see all types of fish and sea creatures when the water recedes well over a hundred yards back.

What are the most important items you have in your carryon and why?

My passport Extra debit/credit card- In case I lose my other one. Backup phone earphones- For Backup Snacks are a must!

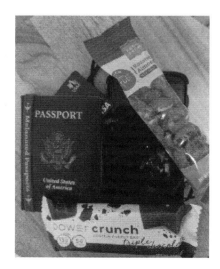

Jerry C' Way

Favorite Calming Beverage or Food to consume while traveling and why?

I always travel with my Yogi Positive Energy tea.

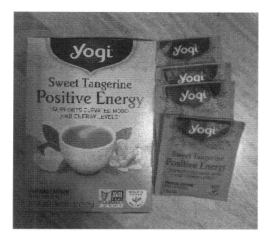

Favorite Calming Music or Audio to listen to while traveling?

Old school music I grew up listening to. Like Keith Sweat. My mama would play his tapes a lot and I knew all of his songs and it takes me back to a happy place in my life.

Favorite Keepsake that keeps you calm or grounded while traveling?

I don't travel with anything that has sentimental value with me in case I lose it. However, every place I visit, I think of each person close to me that I lost and makes me feel as if I'm sharing the experience with them.

What is your most hilarious travel memory?

I've had a lot of hilarious moments while traveling, but one of the funniest one was in Penang, Malaysia. Where this older guy was giving rides on his bicycle with the seat in front. Man, it's so damn hot that day and he had chugged down like 3-4 hot beers. So he's sweating really bad and breathing heavily, so I asked if he wanted me to pedal the bike while he caught his breath. He looked me in my eyes and said please lol. So in short, I paid him to pedal him around town. I still have the video up on my IG with him offering me a hot beer lol.

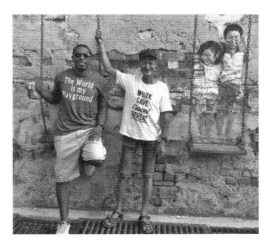

What is your most memorable or touching travel experience?

My most touching travel experience was in India after leaving the Taj Mahal. I got on the wrong train and had to get off at some random stop because my ticket was for a different train company. While waiting I saw a black older gentleman. He was walking with a sheet wrapped around him and had a place where he was sleeping inside the station. So I remember reading about the caste system in India. (Google it if you're not familiar) So there was a stand that sold food, I went and got him something to eat and drink. I also gave him about 2,600 rupees which are only like $40USD. I also gave him the purple outfit and the shoes I wore to the Taj Mahal. This brother never said a word but just hugged me and cried.

What is the worst travel experience you ever had?

Waking up outside of the vehicle we were traveling clueless that I had been ejected and had gone over a cliff. Clueless the gentleman who was sitting next to me who I was laughing and joking with earlier was deceased. *Image of the vehicle on my IG

Favorite Travel Hack?

Scan a copy of your passport and email it to yourself and another family member. Always keep a photocopy of your passport with you in a ziplock bag as well. If it's ever lost or stolen it will help expedite the process at the embassy. Always take an extra phone as a backup in case something happens to your main phone. Most smartphones only need wifi to work.

What is your travel Ritual for keeping calm and maintaining your inner zen?

I just laugh to myself and keep a positive mindset.

Best Travel Tip Advice?

Do not be afraid to travel solo. For the ladies who are on the fence on solo traveling, I would definitely recommend getting a book called "Solo Travel, Try It At Least Once" by Marilene Shane which can be purchased on Amazon

Why is addressing mental health in and self-care with as it relates to people of color so important in the travel community?

We need to break the stigma of mental health being associated with being crazy or simply being ignorant when it comes to discussing or addressing it.

Although we travel often for our mental health, the topic is not emphasized due to shame and stigma. How can we normalize this conversation among the travel communities of color??

We need to discuss it openly more. When I tell my story of my accident and battled with depression, most won't comment publicly but will hit me up privately to tell me they are battling with it and often times ask for help and recommendations. I guess it makes some people more comfortable hearing my story and openly discussing how I've dealt with it.

Jerry C' Way

WEBSITE

TravelFreQk.com

EMAIL

TravelFreQk.@gmail.com

INSTAGRAM HANDLE

TravelFreQk

FACEBOOK PAGE

TravelFreQk

Travel Jokes

Day 147 without sex: I went through the airport metal detector with a fork in my pocket just so someone could feel me up.

CHAPTER 6

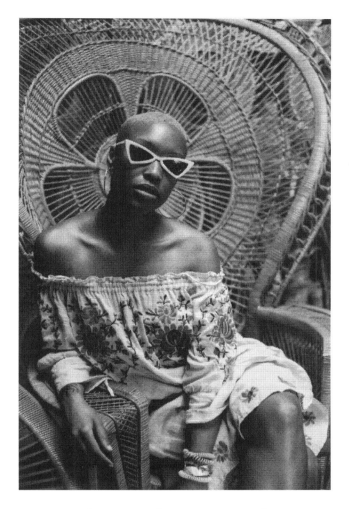

Dana Armstead

Travel n Sh!t Podcast

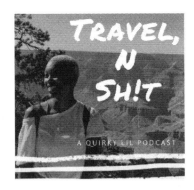

Travel Quote or Travel Mantra you live by
You can learn something from anyone if you ask the right questions.

How has Traveling helped you maintain your mental health as it relates to self-care?

It's something that brings me great joy. I love experiencing myself in these new settings and learning about the people in them. Physically putting myself in beautiful environments and allowing myself to explore the unknown feeds and nurtures what I feel to be the core of my true self. Doing these things that make me happy is self-care for me.

What is your most therapeutic travel destination for stress relief and self-care?

So far I'd say Bali. The massages there are cheap and nature there gave me many opportunities to stop and enjoy the beauty around me. I fondly think back on many "wow" moments that I didn't initially fully appreciate.

What's is the most important items you have in your carryon and why?

I keep a makeup bag full of pills. Pepto, Benadryl, Tylenol, Neosporin, bandaids you name it. Anything I'd take to relieve an ailment at home, I bring with me. I don't want to be abroad and not have something to make sure I'm well enough to enjoy my trip.

Favorite Calming Beverage or Food to consume while traveling and why?

Ginger tea! I especially love it fresh from wherever I am.

Favorite Calming Music or Audio to listen to while traveling?

The Wiz Soundtrack, actually.

Favorite Keepsake that keeps you calm or grounded while traveling?

Unless I'm swimming or wearing different jewelry, I always wear a bracelet and necklace my dad gave me.

What is your most hilarious travel memory?

Traveling to St. Maarten & St. Barths with my mom. We shared so many laughs.

Dana Armstead

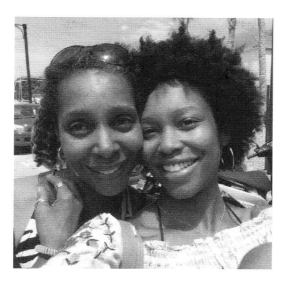

What is your most memorable or touching travel experience?

There are truly so many. I'll go with my time spent in Cartagena, Colombia. I've never felt more appreciated and safe as a black woman. I met incredible people, experienced the diaspora in a new way, and felt so in sync with the universe while I was there. Everything about the people I met and the connections I made were incredible.

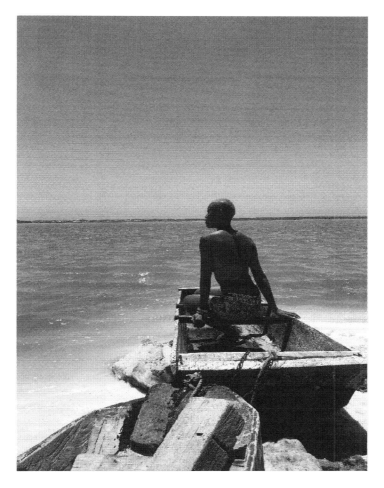

What is the worst travel experience you ever had?

> I decided to go to London with NOTHING planned. When I landed I discovered that I'd overdraft my checking account and I had yet to book my hostel, eat, get train tickets; nothing. Thankfully I had some cash and a credit card on hand, but I'd had a long trip and was at my wit's end by this point. I spent four hours at the airport pretty much crying trying to choose a hostel. By the time I booked it and arrived, I'd lost all motivation to go and see anything. Thankfully for modern technology, I had a friend FaceTime and snap me out of my funk. I spent so much time being depressed, I almost missed out on the few hours I had to explore.

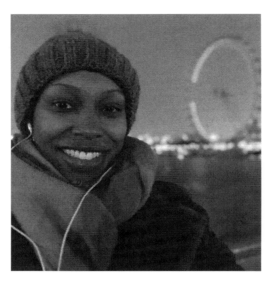

Favorite Travel Hack?

> Packing cubes and app hopping – I never pay the first price I see unless it's the lowest.

What is your travel Ritual for keeping calm and maintaining your inner zen?

> Unpack my fears. What I've learned to do is compare what I'm afraid of at the moment to things I've done that I was initially afraid of. I keep comparing the fear at hand to past fears in an attempt to remind myself through concrete examples that I'm bigger than my fears and I am fully capable of pushing through and conquering them. When I need to calm down and find zen, I consider how important the issue at hand and its associated consequences are to whatever the bigger picture at present is. Will it harm me in any long-term or major way? Have I tried my best? And what's the worst that can happen if I'm wrong? Once I go through those main points I've usually calmed down and realized I'll be fine even if I am wrong about the situation at hand.

Best Travel Tip Advice?

> Go where you can with what you have. It doesn't have to be far or expensive. Just do something meaningful to you, for you.

Why is addressing mental health in and self-care with as it relates to people of color so important in the travel community?

> With social media the way it currently is, it's very easy to get caught up in the most exotic and eye-catching photos. It's easy to get distracted by catching the right angles for photos that we miss a moment. I've personally found it very beneficial to stop and take in as many moments as possible. I purposefully reflect on how I feel and how I am experiencing myself in them. Travel is an experience that presents us with so many opportunities to grow and improve. It's so beneficial to maintaining a strong sense of self to

be able to experience oneself in as many ways and circumstances as possible. In these moments, I think it's important to reflect on issues we have been working on resolving back home in these new environments to get a new set of eyes and fresh perspective on being our best selves.

Although we travel often for our mental health, the topic is not emphasized due to shame and stigma. How can we normalize this conversation among the travel communities of color?

I believe that the more we see and hear of the two being connected, the more normal it will be. If we each do our part by verbalizing the correlation when possible, and by supporting our peers when they too verbalize their own experiences of it, we can make great steps in normalizing the conversation.

WEBSITE

TravelNShitPodcast.com

EMAIL

travelnshitpodcast@gmail.com

INSTAGRAM HANDLE

dCarrie & TravelNShit

FACEBOOK PAGE

www.facebook.com/TravelNShitPodcast

Travel Jokes

Let's skip the Talking stage and go straight to BAECATIONS 🥹
You can tell me yo favorite color and shit on the Plane
✈️🫶❤️🥹

CHAPTER 7

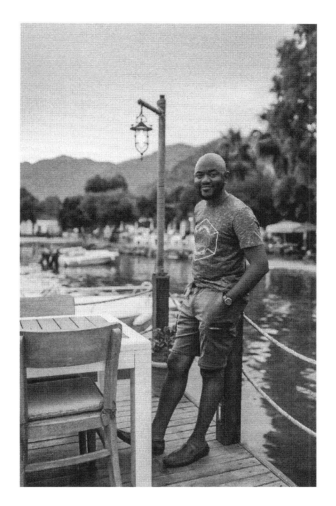

Omoruyi Osagiede

Hey Dip Your Toes In

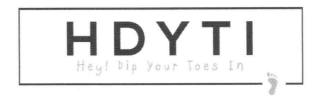

Travel Quote or Travel Mantra you live by
Just dip your toes in the body will follow

How has Traveling helped you maintain your mental health as it relates to self-care?

> Travelling provides a welcome break from routine. Travel, by its very nature, places me in situations where my mind has no other choice but to embrace a whole new environment. This 'escape' from routine offers a chance for introspection, self-awareness, mindfulness and learning.

What is your most therapeutic travel destination for stress relief and self-care?

> The Austrian Alps – Day hiking and spending time outdoors in nature is my happy place. I love the space that the Alps provides and just being around mountains always creates a sense of wonder.

Whats is the most important items you have in your carryon and why?

> Carry on items – Water bottle, protein snacks, gorilla pod (for photos/videos), notebook (for writing).

Favorite Calming Beverage or Food to consume while traveling and why?

> I enjoy port wine and a good bottle of Reisling.

Favorite Calming Music or Audio to listen to while traveling?

> Changes from time to time-based on my mood. Right now I'm enjoying music from Tall Black Guy and Shigeto.

Favorite Keepsake that keeps you calm or grounded while traveling?

> Nothing. I'm not really attached to objects.

What is your most hilarious travel memory?

> I was once mistaken for a Moroccan Berber when, while visiting the Sahara Desert, I dressed up in robes from Northern Nigeria.

Omoruyi Osagiede

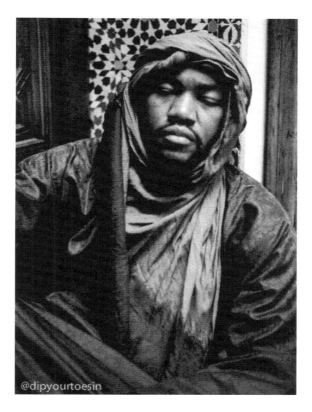

What is your most memorable or touching travel experience?
    Being offered food by total strangers while visiting Bodrum in Turkey recently.

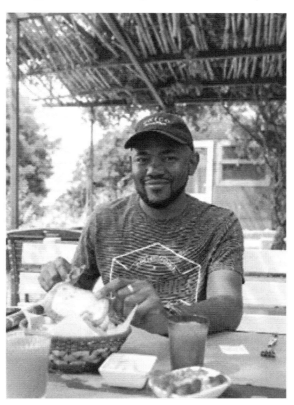

The Ultimate Self-Care Guide for Travelers of Color

What is the worst travel experience you ever had?

One of many. We recently showed up to our 'booked' Airbnb accommodation while visiting Lisbon recently only to find upon arrival, that we had fallen victim to a fake listing on Airbnb. Fortunately, Airbnb was able to refund our money and we ended up finding a penthouse room in Lisbon for the same price.

Favorite Travel Hack?

Avoid airport/travel anxiety. Always leave extra time in your itinerary to get from place to place. Have backup funds available in case you run into trouble.

What is your travel Ritual for keeping calm and maintaining your inner zen?

Deep breathing.

Best Travel Tip Advice?

Consider overnight ferry trips (where they are available). They could save you loads on accommodation and transportation between destinations.

Why is addressing mental health in and self-care with as it relates to people of color so important in the travel community?

The black community traditionally shy's away from the subject of mental health. Young people and men are particularly vulnerable according to recent statistics. I'll narrow this down even further to the black and ethnic minority community. The statistics don't look promising. "People from black and minority ethnic groups living in the UK are more likely to be diagnosed with mental health problems." – MentalHealth.org.uk It is notoriously difficult to find statistics in Nigeria (where I was born) and much of Africa about suicide but I have no doubt that the numbers are equally significant. The Nigerian culture in which I grew up tended to NEVER talk about mental illness (one of the root causes of suicide). When mental illness was ever mentioned, it was usually dismissed as a 'spiritual attack' or 'for weak people' or 'a curse from the person's village'. I was told that men don't cry and that to show any emotion or vulnerability was to show that you 'don't have what it takes' to survive. I was told that people in mental distress were not 'praying hard enough' or needed to 'go see their pastor'. While I cannot claim to be the expert on mental health, I think it's important to acknowledge that none of us is super-human. We all need someone to talk to when we're vulnerable. We are not built to suppress negative thoughts and emotions forever. As black communities who have experienced the mental health benefits that travel can provide, it is important that we share our experiences with our community. People need to know that travel can provide a way out (not an escape from problems that need to be addressed) but rather, a respite and an opportunity to reset, gain perspective and find the strength to face life's many challenges.

Although we travel often for our mental health, the topic is not emphasized due to shame and stigma. How can we normalize this conversation among the travel communities of color?

By talking, sharing, starting conversations and being more open about our personal challenges and victories.

Omoruyi Osagiede

WEBSITE

https://heydipyourtoesin.com

EMAIL

Omoruyi.osagiede@gmail.com

INSTAGRAM HANDLE

dipyourtoesin

FACEBOOK PAGE

HDYTI

Travel Jokes

There are two people in every relationship:

Partner 1: "Okay, I have our passports, boarding passes and car rental reservation"

Partner 2: "Where are we going again?"

CHAPTER 8

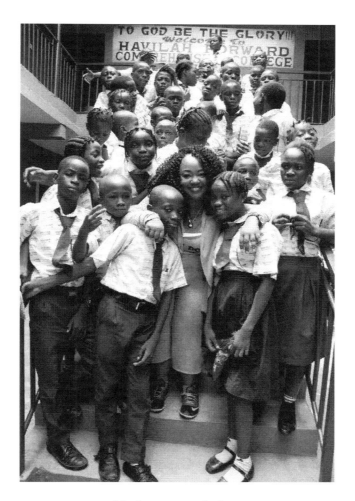

Ejide Fashina

Nigeria Black Out

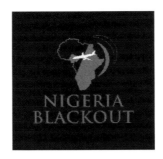

Travel Quote or Travel Mantra you live by

If a man wants to enslave you forever, he will never tell you the truth about your forefathers." – Fela Kuti

Travel Influencer/ Brand Summary

The Nigeria Black Out encourages travelers to experience the buoyant culture, shopping, food, history and exploding art scene in Nigeria. The overall idea of the Nigeria Blackout is to blackout all negative images when it comes to travel/tourism in Nigeria. The Nigeria Blackout shows tourists the overall beauty of the country. Those that visit are encouraged to participate in philanthropy work while visiting the country and walk away feeling empowered

How has Traveling helped you maintain your mental health as it relates to self-care?

Traveling has helped me to maintain my mental health when it relates to self-care because it allows me to disconnect from the everyday hustle and bustle with no specific time limit. Traveling for me gives a different perspective on the world and creates fun challenges. Meeting new people, experiencing different ethnic foods and languages helps me personally to increase my happiness as I am able to do things on my own timing and within my own terms

What is your most therapeutic travel destination for stress relief and self-care?

My most therapeutic travel destination is anywhere that has sun, a beach and a ocean. During my trips to Nigeria, I find so much peace on days where I am able to visit the beach and sit out in the sun and just reflect, relax and listen to the movements of the ocean. There is no better moment than taking in the sun in the country where your ancestors came from.

What are the most important items you have in your carryon and why?

Lysol Spray, Cash on Hand for my destination Personal over-ear headphones, Lysol spray, travel pillow, snacks, refillable water bottle, Nose saline spray, and Doterra Essential Oils

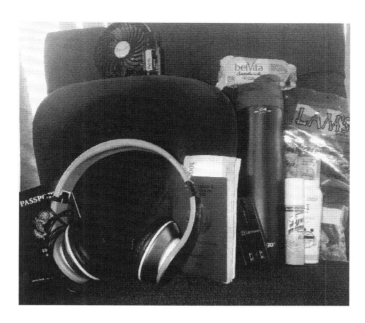

Favorite Calming Beverage or Food to consume while traveling and why?

Starbucks Caramel Frappuccino

Favorite Keepsake that keeps you calm or grounded while traveling?

My cross necklace. I never travel anywhere without it

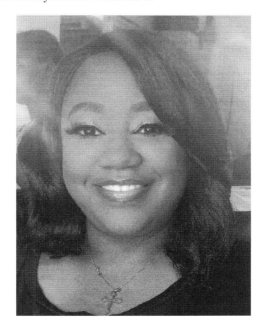

What is your most memorable or touching travel experience?

My most memorable travel experience happened about 20 years ago in Ibadan Nigeria. I was introduced to a lady who prophesized over my life and said that I would do great things and there was a greater purpose in my life than I even knew. At the time I was a teenager and shrugged it over 20 years later I traveled back to the same area and sat at the throne of the Ooni of Ife in Nigeria with the Nigeria Blackout Travel Group and introduced him to our mission of introducing travelers to Nigeria. At that moment it all made sense what the lady 20 years prior was talking about.

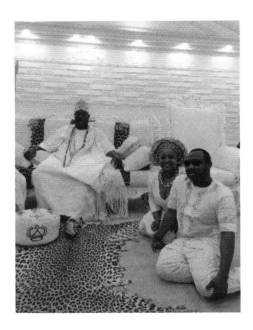

What is the worst travel experience you ever had?

>Missed a flight which caused me to miss cruise ship departure. My luggage went on the flight without me and went to my destination and was already labeled to go on the cruise ship.

Favorite Travel Hack?

>Book flights at least 30 days prior to get the best rates and look at alternate departure and arrival destinations to get good pricing.

What is your travel Ritual for keeping calm and maintaining your inner zen?

>Apply Doterra essential oil to temples of the head and behind ears

Best Travel Tip Advice?

>While traveling be open to experiencing new cultures and places to have the best time.

Why is addressing mental health in and self-care with as it relates to people of color so important in the travel community?

>Mental health is important to address with people of color because mental health issues in the AA community is very taboo to talk about. Most people may not be aware that traveling is a major outlet and can offer some relief when it comes to mental health issues.

Although we travel often for our mental health, the topic is not emphasized due to shame and stigma. How can we normalize this conversation among the travel communities of color?

>We can normalize the conversation in our travel communities by making mental health topics routine discussions. Most dealing with issues are not aware that travel can help and is one of the major ways to practice self-care.

Ejide Fashina

WEBSITE

nigeriablackout.com

EMAIL

ejidefashina@nigeriablackout.com

INSTAGRAM HANDLE

nigeriablackout

FACEBOOK PAGE

https://www.facebook.com/Nigeriablackout/

Travel Jokes

I don't care how many vacations you've seen me on this year. If I say I'm broke, I'm broke.

CHAPTER 9

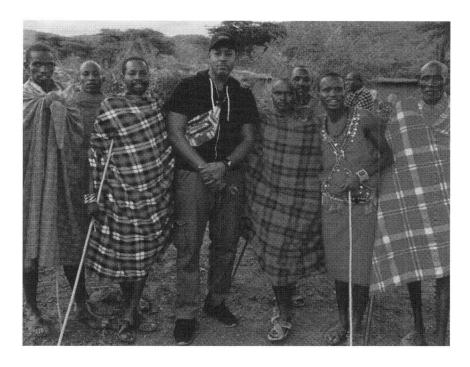

Paul Bashea Williams

Men's Health & International Therapy

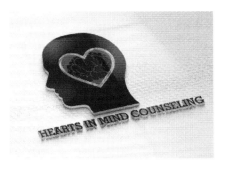

Travel Quote or Travel Mantra you live by
Get away and when you get there; give it away!

Paul Bashea (Bah-Shay) Williams, LCSW-C, LICSW is described as an Intellectual Emotionalist. Someone who understands what a man thinks and how a woman feels. Helping the two meet and have common ground by encouraging emotion and logic to agree. Dedicated father, world traveler, Licensed Mental Health Therapist, Relationship Advisor, Entrepreneur and Author of the book Dear Future Wife: A man's guide and a woman's reference to healthy relationships. He owns and operates his own private practice at Hearts In Mind Counseling where he works with vulnerable youth and specializes in marriage and family, couples, and individual counseling. He travels the world promoting the importance of mental health. Featured on several popular websites, BET, Huffington Post, TV One, Radio One, Fatherly, national syndicated radio shows, ABC, NBC, FOX, CBS, movies, and conferences all over the nation.

How has Traveling helped you maintain your mental health as it relates to self-care?
> It allows me to get away from day to day and explore the lives of others. Opens my eyes to the things I have not seen. A breath of fresh air and calm.

What is your most therapeutic travel destination for stress relief and self-care?
> Africa, it allows me to connect with my history and feels like I can have a fresh start. Being able to walk on the land where everyone comes from is powerful to me.

What is the most important items you have in your carryon and why submit a picture?
> A change of clothes, portable charger, headphones, and my phone.

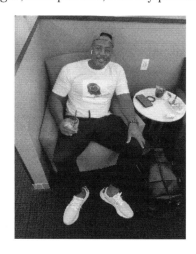

Paul Bashea Williams

Favorite Calming Beverage or Food to consume while traveling and why?

Deep Eddy Vodka with OJ.

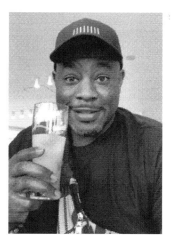

Favorite Calming Music or Audio to listen to while traveling?

Gospel, Samoht, Playa: Cheers 2 U cd, and affirmations

Favorite Keepsake that keeps you calm or grounded while traveling?

A hoodie that allows me to cover my face while traveling when everyone is coughing on the plane or something doesn't smell good.

What is your most hilarious travel memory?

Millie Rocking in Cairo

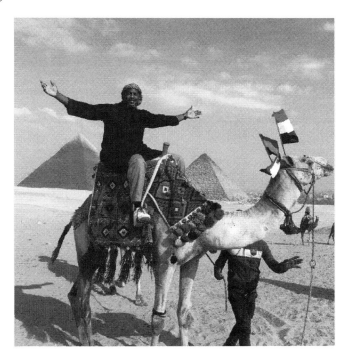

The Ultimate Self-Care Guide for Travelers of Color

What is your most memorable or touching travel experience?

Swimming with sharks in Hawaii or traveling the slums in Kenya

What is the worst travel experience you ever had?

Almost being robbed in Johannesburg.

Favorite Travel Hack?

Staying up the night before so I can sleep the entire flight.

What is your travel Ritual for keeping calm and maintaining your inner zen?

The moment we prepare to take off, I pray. I pray specifically for not just me but also for everyone on the flight. I pray for the pilots and the plane itself. I also pray for other flights everywhere.

Best Travel Tip Advice?

Relax and exercise patience when dealing with those outside of the home and the US.

Why is addressing mental health in and self-care with as it relates to people of color so important in the travel community?

We have to get rid of and address the stigmas of mental health and traveling. Our community sometimes doesn't understand or realize that our community expands past the neighborhoods we live in. The world is huge and important to explore and get connected. Traveling is educational in the book, nature sense but you learn more about yourself when you step outside of your normal routine.

WEBSITE

www.HeartsInMindCounseling.com

EMAIL

Basheawilliams@gmail.com

INSTAGRAM HANDLE

BasheaWilliams

FACEBOOK PAGE

Basheawilliams

Travel Jokes

therapist: so what do we do when we start to feel sad?

me: book another vacay to flex on these hoes.

therapist: no.

CHAPTER 10

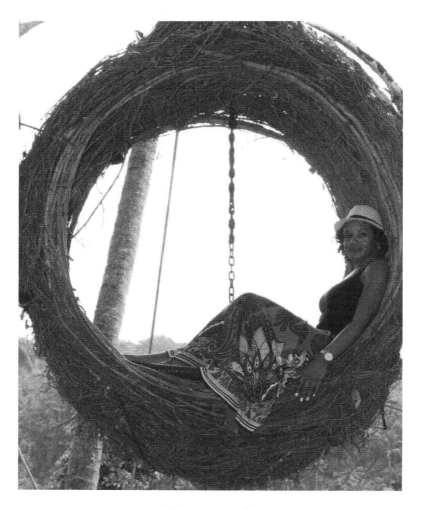

Marilene Shane

"Flying Solo"

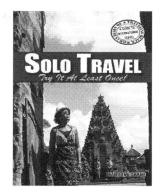

Travel Quote or Travel Mantra you live by

"Traveling alone can be the scariest, most liberating, life-changing experience of your life. Try it at least once." -Anonymous

Travel Influencer/ Brand Summary

Encouraging women to step out of their comfort zones and book a 'solo mission' to conquer fears, challenge limits, and ultimately discover themselves.

How has Traveling helped you maintain your mental health as it relates to self-care?

As a school leader there are times when work and life balance is off, when the feeling of being overwhelmed by the job can seem heavy. I've come to recognize these moments and have begun to use travel as a way to recharge and recalibrate. Solo travel has become the ultimate act of self-care for me. I'm able to come home to myself, quiet the chaos, find my zen and create a game plan for my next steps as I prepare myself to return to the rigor of my work life, with a plan to restore balance.

What is your most therapeutic travel destination for stress relief and self-care?

To date getting to the Continent of Africa has given me the most therapeutic moments of renewal, specifically Zanzibar, Tanzania. The beauty of the people, the landscape, and opportunities to relax and recharge are second to none.

What are the most important items you have in your carryon and why submit a picture?

The most important items in my carryon are my passport, the current book I'm reading, my headsets, sunglasses, snacks and my cell phone.

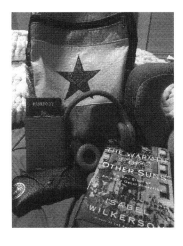

Favorite Calming Beverage or Food to consume while traveling and why?

> My favorite calming beverage whilst traveling is green tea. I moved to Abu Dhabi 5 years ago and tea is a very big deal there, as in most of the world internationally. I've grown to love it in all of its variations. I go so far as to bring some in my bag on most of my solo missions. A nice cup of tea is very relaxing for me.

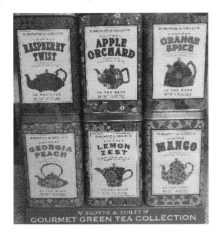

Favorite Calming Music or Audio to listen to while traveling?

> I love anything R-n-B, especially good 90s R-n-B, there's nothing like it. It's just so chill and singers from that time period really could sing. It takes me back to a simpler time in my life, and I know all the words!

Favorite Keepsake that keeps you calm or grounded while traveling?

> I keep a small old school pic of my parents with me when I travel, just a beautiful reminder of my special people when I'm so far away.

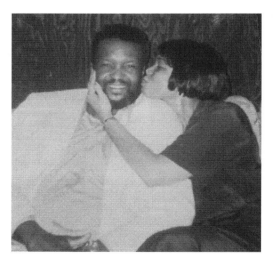

What is your most hilarious travel memory?

> My time in Amsterdam with friends celebrating birthdays. We had the giggles the entire time... ENOUGH SAID!

What is your most memorable or touching travel experience?

> In April 2019 I visited Ghana for the first time. We went to the El Mina Slave Castle in Cape Coast. It was a surreal moment for me, as I feel very driven to learn about my ancestors and feel a deep connection to Africa. We walked through slave dungeons and the Door of No Return and closed out the experience with

a traditional naming ceremony at the point near the water's edge where slaves were loaded on ships headed to the Americas. To be given a name where they lost theirs was the most memorable part of a trip I've ever had. I took a lot of time in quiet reflection on that trip.

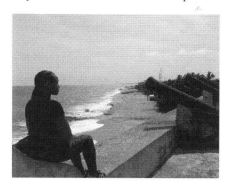

What is the worst travel experience you ever had?

Honestly, I have been blessed to be able to say I haven't had a bad travel experience. All of the many travels I've taken have been amazing, because if nothing else I've learned whilst there about myself or a new location. If I had to pick something, maybe unwanted rain in Thailand when I went in December 2018, but it didn't last long so I'm not sure that counts!

Favorite Travel Hack?

Packing Cubes!! If you like organization and like to have a system for how you pack that also saves room in your bag, you'll love packing cubes. They are amazing!

What is your travel Ritual for keeping calm and maintaining your inner zen?

On every trip, three things are a MUST for my self-care: a scheduled spa day complete with a full body massage and other services, a beach day (I love relaxing by the water), and working out. They both relieve stress in very different ways and allow me to focus some attention on me at my own pace. Every morning I begin the day with a workout, which kicks in those positive, feel-good endorphins, and I'm always certain to get a massage in at some point during my stay to ease away aches and pains and restore calm. I love being by bodies of water and relaxing, and most of my vacations consist of some so I always plan a few days on the beach so i can soak in some good old vitamin D and listen to the water as I nap. So peaceful!

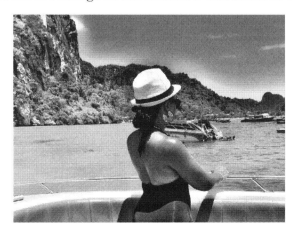

Best Travel Tip Advice?

Plan NOT to plan. So often we plan itineraries out well in advance of our trips without factoring in that we don't know how we will be feeling until we actually get on the trip. When I'm traveling with the purpose of recalibration or to find my zen, I plan NOT to plan. I take each day as it comes. Some days I'll create a full itinerary that has me busy the entire day, other days I literally chill by the pool and relax all day. The key is I don't make those decisions until I get there, so there's no pressure to do or not to do, I'm just taking each day as it comes. Those kinds of trips are liberating. Freedom feels good!

Why is addressing mental health in and self-care with as it relates to people of color so important in the travel community?

Although we travel often for our mental health, the topic is not emphasized due to shame and stigma. How can we normalize this conversation among the travel communities of color?

There are tons of online Black Travel groups who discuss so many topics around travel. I think if we start having these conversations there and at meetups and travel conferences people would begin to feel more comfortable with conversations about mental health and the benefits of travel on it.

WEBSITE

www.diaryofblackwomentravlers.com

EMAIL

mshane3723@gmail.com

INSTAGRAM HANDLE

@wander_lene

FACEBOOK PAGE

Marilene Shane

Travel Jokes

Flying Spirit Airlines right now. The flight attendant just said "To all of you that said you'd never fly Spirit Airlines again... Welcome back"

CHAPTER 11

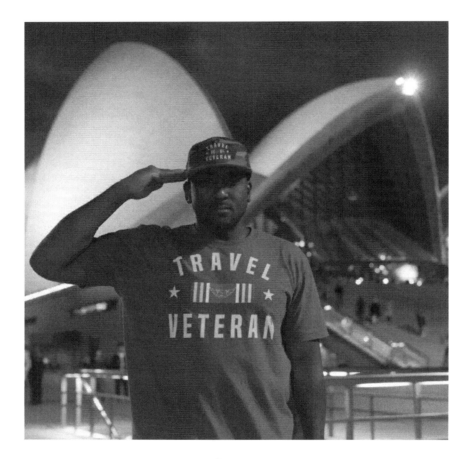

Kurtis Henry

Black Military Veterans & Travel
Runway Boyz Part 1

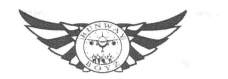

Travel Quote or Travel Mantra you live by

Runway Boyz "We're International"
Traveling is medicine for mental health

Travel Influencer/ Brand Summary

The Runway Boyz Flight Club is a clothing company, representing the traveling lifestyle. Founded in 2005, The Runway Boyz started as a group of active duty Air Force members, making a point to get together at least twice per year, no matter where in the world. By adding new members with each trip, and traveling the globe together, The Runway Boyz became a lifestyle. Using their international connections, the group would start producing clothing for men, women and children in late 2012.

The Flight Travel Group was started in 2014, by retired U.S. military veteran, Kurtis H. He wanted to create a haven for new and old travelers, to see the world, without having to worry about planning. By organizing vacations, travel, and sharing details of places traveled, the vision of an international travel group, has come to fruition.

How has Traveling helped you maintain your mental health as it relates to self-care?

Traveling has helped with my anxiety and depression in a way that no pill ever could. It has allowed me to relieve stress even if it is for a short period of time. Having that break from my normal routine helps relieve the anxiety from doing the things that I am obligated to do on a normal basis. Self-care and relaxation are important in regards to mental and physical health because you only have one body and it wasn't meant to be working constantly without any fulfillment or satisfaction. I truly believe that travel also allows you to develop a stronger mind as you experience new things and view situations from different perspectives.

What is your most therapeutic travel destination for stress relief and self-care?

There a few places that I enjoy visiting. If I need a quick vacation, I would choose the Caribbean. When I visit Jamaica, I don't need many plans. Just give me the beach in Negril, Montego Bay, or Ochos Rios with a plate of Jerk Chicken and I'm in heaven. If I'm looking for an outdoor adventure on a quick trip, I would pick Costa Rica. I loved zip-lining, rafting and horseback riding. The country is a nature lovers paradise. I never knew I liked the outdoors as much until I went there. I plan on going back to visit Manuel Antonio national park and visit the Caribbean side of the country. Most people know me from my trips to Brazil. I frequently visit Brazil and I stay in the country for at least a third of the year. Salvador Bahia and Rio de Janeiro are where I spend most of my time but I tend to go off the beaten path to cities and other states within Brazil that see very few Americans.

Whats is the most important items you have in your carryon and why?

A pen, power cords, passport, toiletries, change of underwear, my drone, mobile wifi box, GoPro and universal plug for charging.

Favorite Calming Beverage or Food to consume while traveling and why?

A Greek meat variety plate or Jerk Chicken

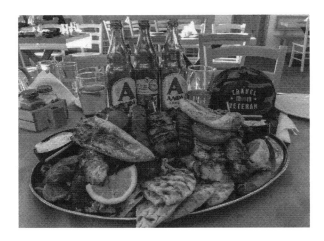

Favorite Calming Music or Audio to listen to while traveling?

> Eclectic hip hop, jazz hip hop fusion, Brazilian Samba and Pagode

Favorite Keepsake that keeps you calm or grounded while traveling?

> My camera roll keeps me calm while I'm traveling. During flights, my anxiety and impatience tend to spike. When I go back and view photos and videos from previous trips, this helps calms my nerves and keeps my mind occupied

What is your most hilarious travel memory?

> The most hilarious moment in travel I have had was also a fun one. I did the OZ jet boats in Sydney. They are boats that zip around Sydney Harbour and do all kinds of crazy spins and turns. The whole boat was holding on for dear life while the driver did all types of tricks in his high-speed boat. I was in the front row letting all the adrenaline kick in while laughing the whole time.

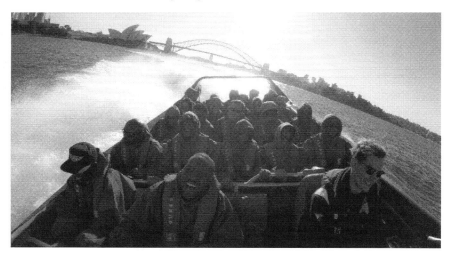

What is your most memorable or touching travel experience?

> My most memorable experience has to be my first soccer game in Brazil. Immediately became a fan of Flamengo of Rio De Janeiro.

Kurtis Henry

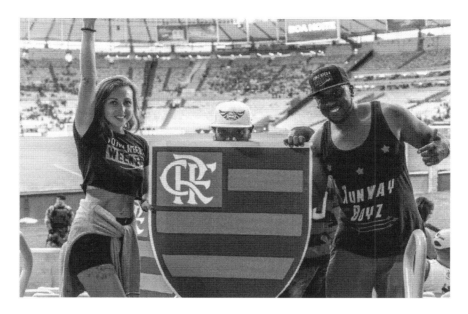

What is the worst travel experience you ever had?

    I received some bad travel advice about a city on the island of Crete. I was 28 at the time. When I went there were nothing but teenagers there and all the bars were serving fake alcohol. I was ready to go in the first 24 hours.

Favorite Travel Hack?

    Sometimes booking an international flight starting at a major airport like LAX or NYC and buying another ticket to that major airport from your starting point can be cheaper than buying the whole international ticket together that starts at a smaller airport that is closer to you.

What is your travel Ritual for keeping calm and maintaining your inner zen?

    Flying my drone and filming my vacations helps me keep calm. I love doing amateur cinematography. Its a hobby and my favorite way to preserve the memories of my travels.

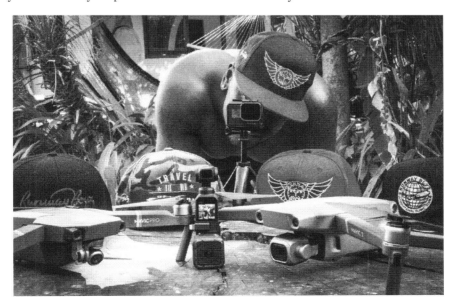

Best Travel Tip Advice?

Travel at least once a year. It does not have to be international. Just get away from your regular surroundings for a few days when you can.

Why is addressing mental health in and self-care with as it relates to people of color so important in the travel community?

Mental health should be important to people of color because it can affect your physical health. This can lead to serious health conditions and even death. Bad health and traveling don't mix. Unfortunately, I have heard of travelers that have died while on vacation due to bad health conditions. Your health is your wealth!

Although we travel often for our mental health, the topic is not emphasized due to shame and stigma. How can we normalize this conversation among the travel communities of color?

We all have our problems. People post travel pictures and blogs that only show the good times in their life. Life is not always positive so it is important to address mental issues when the symptoms occur. We live in a society of high expectations. This can lead to anxiety and depression. Discussing mental health helps those who have little experience with these issues identify what to look for in their personal lives. Some people may suffer and may not even be aware. We can also help each other with resources while at home or suggest places to travel to that may specialize in mental, spiritual, and physical relaxation.

Travel Jokes

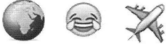

Worrying you've accidentally packed 4 kilos of cocaine and a dead goat as you walk through 'nothing to declare' at the airport.

CHAPTER 11
CONTINUED

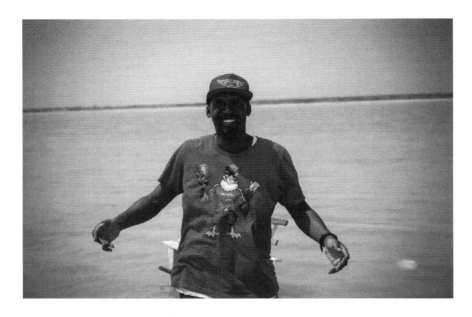

Jakarri Stroman

Runway Boyz Part II

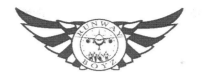

Travel Quote or Travel Mantra you live by
I'd rather die living reckless than of boredom

How has Traveling helped you maintain your mental health as it relates to self-care?

Traveling has always been a cleansing experience for me. I suffer from anxiety and depression. Usually at home, I'm at work or I'm at home. I'm almost a recluse in the physical form and mentally with friends and family. Forget about social interactions.... That all changes the moment I start packing for the next adventure. I'm happy, smiling, excited to get out and about. Once I land, I'm chatting up with everyone I see, trying every new food, learning about the local culture, and having new experiences. It's like night and day for me. When I get home, reflecting on the trip usually helps me cope better as well. I tend to learn something about myself on each vacation that helps me internally. I don't know where I would be if I was trapped by the boundaries of my state.

What is your most therapeutic travel destination for stress relief and self-care?

Rio De Janeiro, Brazil is top of my list. I've traveled to 5 continents and haven't found a place quite like it. It's right by the beach for relaxation or the rain forest for exploration. You have a major city with everything that comes with, but also mountains to climb 15 minutes away, and sprawling neighborhoods on the other side. The people really make it welcoming. For everything we see on TV, it's nothing like that with the gangs and violence. Everyone I met has been welcoming and very helpful. They won't give you directions, they'll walk with you there. The prices on everything is cheap from accommodations to the food to excursions to nightlife. And the nightlife is amazing. 7 days of the week, there will be a host of parties, samba parties, clubs, and events, that last until the sun comes up. I always know if I need to relax and take some time to myself, I can get away to Rio and get everything I need.

Whats is the most important items you have in your carryon and why?

My camera and my drone. I make sure to carry them on every flight because I take thousands of pictures on vacation. I couldn't imagine if they got lost or stolen. That's another helpful item because taking people's pictures, and asking permission first, is a huge step for me in breaking my social interaction issues.

Favorite Calming Beverage or Food to consume while traveling and why?

Water!! I never drink enough water at home (nor walk). But I get more than enough on vacation from being outside all day, usually in hot weather, and walking around the city. We all should be drinking more water, but you really see the difference on vacation. I actually feel better after a week of no soda and juice products

Favorite Calming Music or Audio to listen to while traveling?

Jakarri! Shameless plug, I know! I write most of my music while traveling. I'm not a mumble rapper or even one all about lying and stunting. I write about my mental issues, my life, my feelings. My writing is therapeutic so it's not surprising most is written while away. I also shoot most of my video on vacation, so I can splice it up with exotic locations and topics.

Favorite Keepsake that keeps you calm or grounded while traveling?

My daughter passed away 2 years ago. I have a keychain with her name on it that only leaves the house for vacation. I feel like I take her everywhere and she'll watch over me.

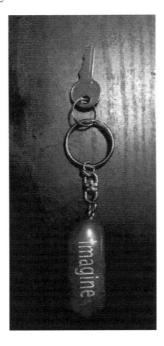

What is your most hilarious travel memory?

I went to the tiger sanctuary in Thailand. I knew I wasn't going to handle the big tigers so I got in with two babies. These guys were WILD!! With claws and teeth big enough to hurt, but too young to sedate. Watching them roll around, play, fight and take pics was so much fun.

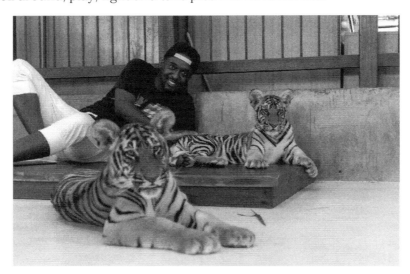

What is your most memorable or touching travel experience?

My second trip to Rio. The first time, my best friend had to cancel about 3 weeks before we left. I went anyway and was alone, knew no Portuguese, but managed to have an OK time. The second time, I went with about 15 people. That was an event for the ages. My first time falling in love with Rio.

Jakarri Stroman

What is the worst travel experience you ever had?

Croatia for the Fresh Island 3 day Festival. The country was absolutely beautiful. The problem was the festival. Every single artist canceled. The forest next to the venue caught on fire so shows got canceled for the replacements. The problem was, you wouldn't find out until 8pm the night of. Nothing was done for any of the guests either. So essentially I came all the way there to be let down daily.

Favorite Travel Hack?

Not sure if it's a hack, but always look for an Airbnb first. The money saved on cooking, with the added space and having your own home, is always worth it. And if you have more than 2 people, it'll be cheaper then a hotel

What is your travel Ritual for keeping calm and maintaining your inner zen?

Tell myself, "That's nothing but fear talking" Helps me get past 99% of things that are truly nothing more than your head telling you to be scared.

Best Travel Tip Advice?

Find the locals and ask them for their reviews on things you want to see/eat/do. They live there every day. They have a better grasp than any traveler, articles or reviews.

Why is addressing mental health in and self-care with as it relates to people of color so important in the travel community?

It's important because it simply is not addressed as much as it should be in our community. There's still a stigma that it's not a medical issue. That people are either "crazy" or "normal" and that medicine, therapy and mental health are not to be discussed or entertained. That is a recipe for disaster as this affects all races and colors.

Although we travel often for our mental health, the topic is not emphasized due to shame and stigma. How can we normalize this conversation among the travel communities of color?

I think as the younger generation grows, they'll help to normalize things. We are getting to a point where "get over it" and "man up" isn't working anymore. And kids who grew up with mental health problems, are now having kids, with mental health problems. It's a shame we can't seem to get the older generation to buy-in. I would hope that as time goes on, their kids and grandkids will be able to help them open up and embrace the conversation at least

WEBSITE

RunwayBoyz.com

Flightlifegroup.com

EMAIL

therunwayboyz@gmail.com

INSTAGRAM HANDLE

@jakarri_rwb

@therunwayboyz

@flightlifegroup

FACEBOOK PAGE

https://www.facebook.com/FlightLifeGroup/

https://www.facebook.com/TheRunwayBoyz/

Travel Jokes

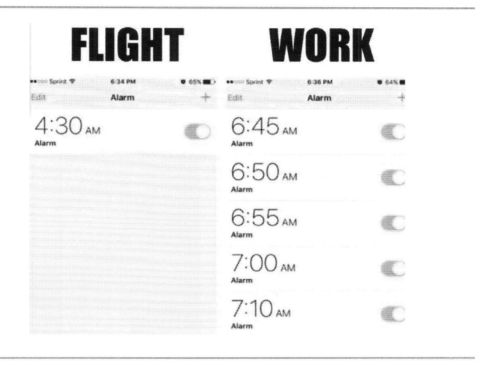

CHAPTER 12

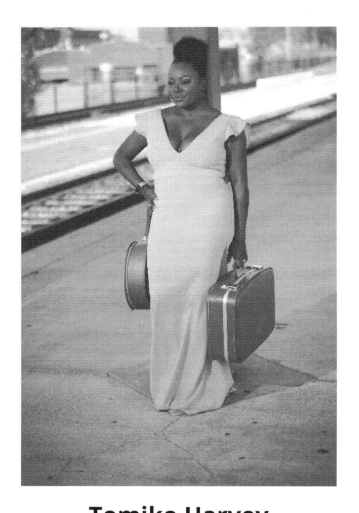

Tomiko Harvey

It's all about Passports & Grub

PASSPORTS & GRUB

Travel Quote or Travel Mantra you live by
The goal is to die with memories not dreams
so I explore the world now

Travel Influencer/ Brand Summary

A wanna be nomadic traveler but otherwise a Tennessee based Digital Marketer where I inspire African American families to travel more whether its a weekend trip to the Smoky Mountains or across the globe to Rome. My readers will find resources to help them seek out culture and adventure in every destination.

How has Traveling helped you maintain your mental health as it relates to self-care??

Travel helps on an interpersonal growth level as well; seeing different people and cultures and encountering them directly as individuals and human beings opens yourself to becoming more tolerant and flexible about unfamiliar ways of life. Travel for me is a break from stressors piled up at home and is an escape where I can focus on what makes me happy. The change of pace helps reduce my body's stress hormone and even when I return home, the memories of my last destination will help maintain a "zen space" I can revisit whenever I need to escape mentally.

What is your most therapeutic travel destination for stress relief and self-care?

Costa Rica is the place I go in mind when I am stressed by the people, the food, to the sense of community and family. Costa Rica has everything one needs when it comes to self-care and also the country focus is not on material things but focuses more on health and community and you can sense that when interacting with the locals. Costa Rica is amazing!

What's is the most important items you have in your carryon and why?

Phone Charger! Whew Lawd don't let me forget my charger

Favorite Calming Beverage or Food to consume while traveling and why?

I love Seafood so any type of pasta seafood just fills my heart with joy!

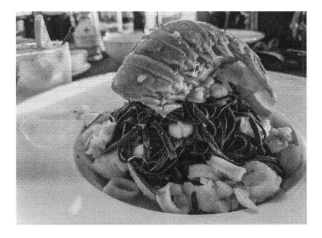

Favorite Calming Music or Audio to listen to while traveling?

I listen to "The Secret" it puts me in a positive space and reminds me of my words and attitude matter.

Favorite Keepsake that keeps you calm or grounded while traveling?

My brother Marco died of complications from High Blood pressure at a very young age so he is always with me and in my heart.

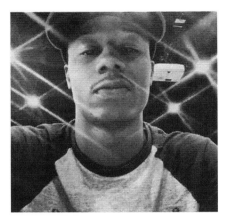

What is your most hilarious travel memory?

My hubby eating termites in the jungles of Belize. They taste like chicken!

What is your most memorable or touching travel experience?

My husband James and I were Rome a few years ago and after a day of walking and taking in Rome we were starving. The restaurant where we wanted to have dinner had a line wrapped around the building with a 2-hour wait. Clearly, I had to find another alternative and right across the street from the busy restaurant was a completely empty restaurant with a little old man standing on the curb as people walked buy his restaurant without giving him a second thought. The hubby and I decided we were tired and just need to eat. This turned out to be one of the best decisions I've ever made when it came to food. OMG! My meal was simple just pasta and clams but the pasta was like butter and melted in my mouth with every bite and the little old man saw my expressions with every bite and his face just lit up. He couldn't speak English and I couldn't speak Italian but we had this moment in time where we were the only two people in the world. The little old man grabbed my face and kissed my cheeks. It felt like the world actually stopped and my husband calls him my grandpa because of the connection we had that one day in Rome and I often think about him and wonder if he is still alive.

What is the worst travel experience you ever had?

I didn't enjoy Belize. While the country is beautiful the people are extremely poor and I felt "privileged" to be in a country enjoying the beauty of its resources while the people are living in such dire conditions. I left their feeling a bit depressed.

Favorite Travel Hack?

Be nice! Be nice to the flight attendants, be nice to the hotel staff, be nice to your waiters and waitress. It pays to be nice because you never know if you will get upgraded which is exactly what happened to the hubby and I on our way to Jamaica. The flight was delayed due to weather and everybody was giving the flight crew a hard time and we sat there and talked to the crew and never complained. Once we boarded we were upgraded to first class. My favorite hack is just to be nice.

Tomiko Harvey

What is your travel Ritual for keeping calm and maintaining your inner zen?

I don't really get upset when traveling. If I get lost I just turn around, if my flight is delayed I take a nap, my food isn't prepared properly I order something else. Things will happen but it is your attitude that determines how you will allow mishaps to affect you. Have a cocktail and keep it moving.

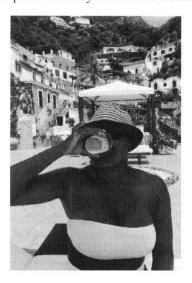

Best Travel Tip Advice?

Travel with an open mind and interact with the locals and understand their culture.

Why is addressing mental health in and self-care with as it relates to people of color so important in the travel community?

A person of color comes with a lot of generational baggage. Although we use travel as an alternative therapy tool, we have deeper issues that must be unpacked by professionals. Those issues won't be resolved by one trip

Although we travel often for our mental health, the topic is not emphasized due to shame and stigma. How can we normalize this conversation among the travel communities of color?

I have been in therapy for 20 years and I have never been ashamed that I need therapy so for me telling people that it is ok to ask for help. Traveling is a therapy for me and we as a community have to be open to the idea but that only comes from people like you and myself saying out loud it's ok

WEBSITE

www.passportsandgrub.com

EMAIL

passportsandgrubs@gmail.com

INSTAGRAM HANDLE

https://www.instagram.com/passportsandgrub/

FACEBOOK PAGE

https://www.facebook.com/passportsandgrub/T

Travel Jokes

It's always a "wyd" text, it's never a "I booked you an all inclusive trip to the Virgin Islands because you said you was craving seafood" 😒.

CHAPTER 13

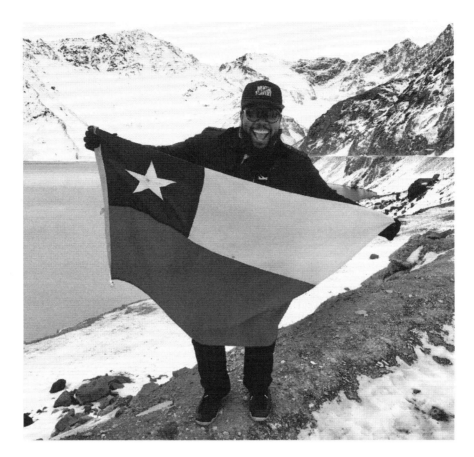

Brian Oliver

Beyond Bmore

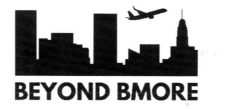

BEYOND BMORE

Travel Quote or Travel Mantra you live by
"Go By Yourself!"

How has Traveling helped you maintain your mental health as it relates to self-care?

Travel is a form of therapy for me. I often sit on the plane and just meditate, brainstorm and recuperate. My best ideas come to mind often while flying and relaxing. Many of the destinations I have visited have also put me in a place of peace that was indescribable. I encourage others to travel as much as possible not just for leisure but for mental health and wellness.

What is your most therapeutic travel destination for stress relief and self-care?

Anywhere with of view of the city/country has proven to be therapeutic for stress relief and self-care. Just relaxing on a rooftop/balcony and gathering my thoughts has helped me tremendously in the past.

Whats is the most important items you have in your carryon and why?

My Bose noise-canceling headphones. They allow me to eliminate outside noise and listen to my music of choice at the moment. Often, I am not listening to anything, but the silence is relaxing and helpful in thinking and planning.

Favorite Calming Beverage or Food to consume while traveling and why?

A well-made cocktail also helps.

Favorite Calming Music or Audio to listen to while traveling?

R&B

Favorite Keepsake that keeps you calm or grounded while traveling?

My most hilarious travel memory would be hiking a mountain in Chile while underdressed and freezing. There were snow and ice all over and I can't count the number of times I fell during the hour's long trek up and down

What is your most memorable or touching travel experience?

My most memorable and touching travel experience was volunteering at a school in the Kibera slums of Nairobi, Kenya. The time spent with the kids there was amazing. I returned again and volunteered for a few more days during a later visit.

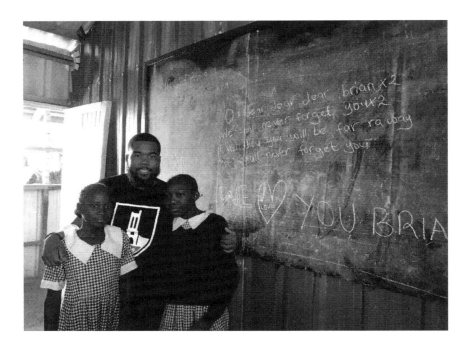

What is the worst travel experience you ever had?

My worse travel experience was during a trip to Bali in 2017. The Volcano began to smoke and I was stranded on the island for extra days trying to get to Japan. I missed all of my connecting flights home and had to pay a large amount of money to eventually get back to Baltimore.

Favorite Travel Hack?

I have been able to travel on many first and business class flights thanks to learning a lot of information on points and miles. It has changed the way I travel.

What is your travel Ritual for keeping calm and maintaining your inner zen?

I often force myself to stay in my hotel room and rest/sleep, even if I have plans. Once I do this I find myself recharged and calm if there had been any previous issues.

Best Travel Tip Advice?

Know which websites to follow and subscribe to that post deals 24/7. Do not hesitate when a great fare appears! They sell out or cancel quickly and every minute counts.

Why is addressing mental health in and self-care with as it relates to people of color so important in the travel community?

Many people in the travel community simply travel to escape things that they never address. Doing so never solves anything and the issues remain. It is important to know that while traveling can be a form of therapy, it may not always solve the problems we face. Being free from mental illness and unhealthy thoughts is crucial to our wellbeing and lives of others around us.

Although we travel often for our mental health, the topic is not emphasized due to shame and stigma. How can we normalize this conversation among the travel communities of color?

We must begin to openly discuss mental health not just in private conversation but in our various online communities and groups. We have been taught forever as people of color that mental illness does not

Brian Oliver

exist for us. This is simply untrue. While we neglect these issues we are further harming ourselves and our quality of life. We must take the same actions that others do and heal/grow.

WEBSITE

www.beyondbmore.com

EMAIL

brian@beyondbmore.com

INSTAGRAM HANDLE

@beyondbmore

FACEBOOK PAGE

www.facebook.com/beyondbmore

Travel Jokes

Whoever brings the friend that's not my friend on the trip that ruins the trip you're responsible for that friend.

CHAPTER 14

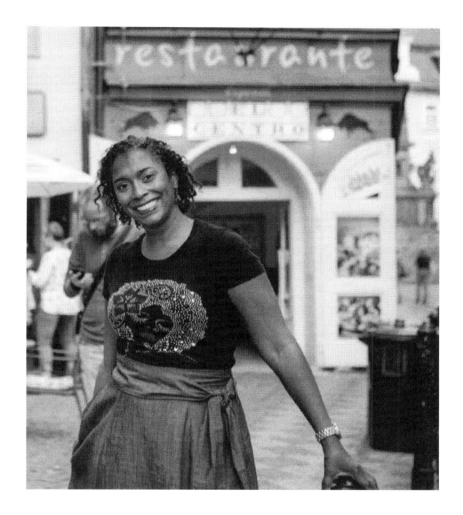

La Tessa Montgomery

Let me buy you drank

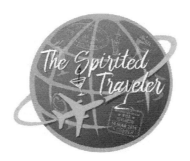

Travel Quote or Travel Mantra you live by

"Not all who wander are lost."- J.R.R. Tolkien "Traveling- it leaves you speechless, then turns you into a storyteller." -Ibn Battuta

Travel Influencer/ Brand Summary

The Spirited Traveler was born out of my combined loves of exploring and tasty cocktails. As The Spirited Traveler, I showcase & promote diversity in the worlds of traveling and bespoke cocktails & spirits

How has Traveling helped you maintain your mental health as it relates to self-care?

Traveling puts me directly in touch with a side of myself that just can't be negative. This side doesn't fret, doesn't worry about the tedium, doesn't wallow in hurt feelings, broken hearts, or disappointments. When traveling, I'm free to be in wonder, free to live in the now, free to explore my creatively, and most importantly, free to reflect on my life and all the blessings I have.

What is your most therapeutic travel destination for stress relief and self-care?

Since I travel to a new place each year on my big adventures, I don't have a place I repeatedly visit for stress relief and self-care. However, I will say, I absolutely cannot wait to visit both Paris and Italy again. There's something about the vibe of Paris: the sights, the smell, the sounds, the art, that makes me long to walk the streets and take in the slices of life I happen upon. And Italy is full of beauty, the sun, and the sea. That, in itself, is the perfect prescription for distressing. Not to mention the wonderful food and wine at your fingertips. As an author, I enjoy places that stimulate my creativity and allow me to use my experiences in my writing. Both Paris and Italy serve as bottomless bowls of creative energy for me, feeding my imagination and helping me gain clarity.

Whats is the most important items you have in your carryon and why?

LOL- I'm actually in the process of writing an article on carrying on essentials. If I have to pick one thing as my most important, I will have to say my earphones. I need peace and the ability to zone out while on long flights and I am not always in the mood the chat to other passengers. Being able to tune out ambient noises and enjoying movies, audiobooks, or music on flights keeps me happy.

La Tessa Montgomery

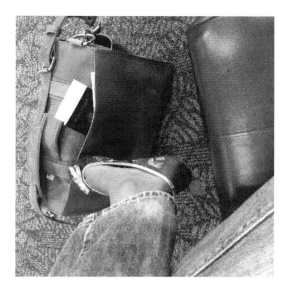

Favorite Calming Beverage or Food to consume while traveling and why?

I don't know about calming, but I do enjoy a nice glass of wine while in flight. Enjoying a glass, or 2, is part of my inflight routine before I settle in for my nap. Here's a pic of champagne Delta Airlines so graciously provided on a recent trip to Italy.

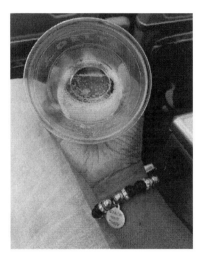

Favorite Calming Music or Audio to listen to while traveling?

I have a playlist I created of all of my favorite songs, regardless of genre, titled "Good Music". This is my go-to playlist I listen to while traveling. Now, my friends will tell you my taste in music is highly questionable, but it works for me. 😊

Favorite Keepsake that keeps you calm or grounded while traveling?

I've never really considered this question before. I don't have keepsakes I travel with, per se. But I will say, I can't be without my earphones when I'm traveling. I rely on them for my music and for directions. I listen to music nearly nonstop, especially when I am traveling solo. I love adding new memories and emotions to my favorite songs, gained by exploring new cities and cultures while my fav tunes are playing in my ear. It's a nice way for me to extend my trip when I return and a great way to take me back to a place or time when I need a bit of a mental break. I will always remember John Mayer's "Clarity" playing while I sat out a cafe in Prague contemplating the next phase of my life. Likewise, I remember what was playing when I took the train from Rome to Naples, when I visited the Trevi Fountain, as I walked in the rain in Florence.... I could go on, but I think you get the picture-lol.

What is your most hilarious travel memory?

Trying to get to Versailles from Paris via train. OMG, this was an experience. Long story short, I'd read and researched how to get to Versailles from Paris taking the train. Now, but this time, I'd been in Paris for close to 3 days, and thought I was an expert at using the Metro. This proved to NOT be the case. So, what I failed to catch in my many hours of research was I needed to go to the actual train station to transfer, NOT catch another Metro train. So, after going back to the metro station (and using up tickets each time) to look for this fictional train to Versailles several times, to encountering the most non-helpful and friendly train station attendant, to wandering around a French neighborhood at 7 am when NOTHING is open and no one spoke English.... I had to play a highly amusing game of charades with a group of young people so we could understand each other and get to the right spot. Once at the train station, my travel companion and I promptly busted out laughing the

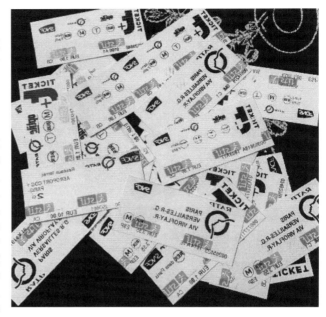

shenanigans we'd just been through. I've attached a picture that shows a lot of the Metro tickets I brought back with me. If you look closely, you will be able to make out several (way more than was actually needed) that say Versailles

What is your most memorable or touching travel experience?

My most touching travel experience.... I'd have to say my visit to the Vatican left me speechless and impressed me more than I thought it would. The history, the art, the sheer size of it blew me away. Getting the see The Sistine Chapel ceiling person is a memory I hope I never lose. Pictures are not allowed, so I will have to rely on the internet and my memory to relive that one. But overall, I was deeply affected by the beauty of all the art, the craftsmanship is just beyond. And St. Peters.... there are no words to succinctly sum the reverence, grandeur, and scale of that church. I remember letting the tour move on a bit just so I could stand (in relative peace) and take it all in.

What is the worst travel experience you ever had?

Fortunately for me, I've not had a majorly bad travel experience. However, I can say getting lost for hours in Venice recently was not fun. At all. I had a planned tour I'd put together all ready to go. But I quickly realized once I stepped outside the train station, that I was not prepared for the

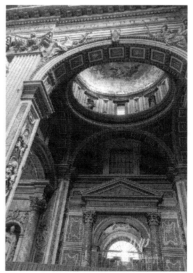

overwhelming feeling of otherness I would get in Venice. The city doesn't look or feel like any other place I'd ever been, and the second I turned down a random street in search of San Marco's I was hopelessly lost. It took me over 2 hours to find my way back to the train station and I don't think I'd ever been more afraid while traveling solo in my life. I encountered troubles with the language barriers and the fact the street names are just not very visible over there. Not to mention, I had no wifi at the time, so my trusty map was a no go. I wandered and wandered, and wandered around that city with its tiny streets and imposing buildings (that look very familiar). And after buying an actual map (which was of absolutely no help at all-lol), and literally stopping by every third shop or restaurant I passed, I got back to the train station. So after I'd calmed down and gotten myself together, I snapped a couple of photos and went in to wait on my train. In fact, the pic I've attached with this story is the one I took of myself, by accident, as I was trying to fold up my useless map. I look quite unhappy-lol It's funny now, my level of panic at the time was not.

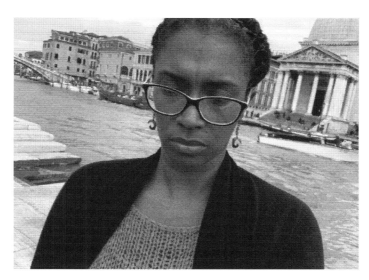

Favorite Travel Hack?

Using SkyScanner.net to pre-price my flights and get an idea of when I will arrive and leave my destination. Once I get this, I start competitively pricing flights and planning my travel itinerary.

What is your travel Ritual for keeping calm and maintaining your inner zen?

Music, a glass of wine, and an outdoor seat so I can people watch. This is my favorite mid-day and early evening activities. I've worked on taking breaks daily on my trips now. I use to just hit the ground hard and pound it until I got back home. After straining my calf muscle in Prague, I no longer do that. I always find it relaxing to chill with a glass of the country's specialty and people watch. This affords me the headspace to zone out and listen to the sounds of the city, my heart, & poke at my subconscious a little.

Best Travel Tip Advice?

I have two travel advice/travel tips articles up on my site, and I have to say, I'm torn between two to say is my best travel advice: 1) Have fun and enjoy yourself 2) Prepare a travel itinerary, no matter how loose or detailed it is. Even if you decide to completely toss it out once you land, at least you have it if you need it.

Why is addressing mental health in and self-care with as it relates to people of color so important in the travel community?

I love traveling and visiting new places. However, I noticed I didn't see many people that looked like me on my adventures: a youngish middle-aged, African American, female, solo traveler. Although it initially sounds like freedom, it can also trigger depression and anxiety because people of color go through so mu

Although we travel often for our mental health, the topic is not emphasized due to shame and stigma. How can we normalize this conversation among the travel communities of color?

I say just have the conversations. If you talk about it publicly, eventually others will come to accept it. It's how most trends are adopted. Someone with no fear of judgment how does care what others think will step out, either in a new fashion or on a new or unpopular platform to state their beliefs and feelings. This tends to encourage those that feel the same to adapt and move in the current with the trailblazer.

WEBSITE

www.TheSpirited-Traveler.com

EMAIL

GetSpirited@TheSpirited-Traveler.com

INSTAGRAM HANDLE

TheSpirited_Traveler

FACEBOOK PAGE

The Spirited Traveler

Travel Jokes

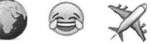

Why do people ask "how was work?"

Like, work is work...I would rather be in Europe right now, naked on a yacht, while destroying my liver...

...but here I am.

CHAPTER 15

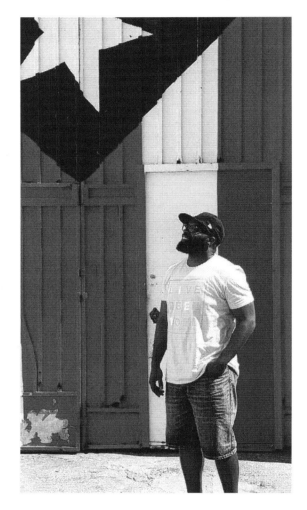

Akeem Tolson

Mr. Puerto

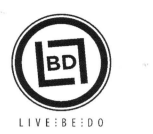

LIVE : BE : DO

Travel Quote or Travel Mantra you live by
Live. Be. Do.

Travel Influencer/ Brand Summary

We encourage people to achieve the highest quality of life regardless of any perceived obstacles.

How has Traveling helped you maintain your mental health as it relates to self-care?

Traveling allows me to step away from my regular routine. I'm self-employed. There were times in the past when I would work myself to the point of burnout. After a few instances of mental/ physical exhaustion, I figured there was really no point in working that hard if I didn't play just as hard. I decided that I'd earned the right to plan regular trips as mental health breaks.

What is your most therapeutic travel destination for stress relief and self-care?

Puerto Rico has become my place of peace. It has the look and feel of a faraway, international destination without the hassle of US Customs and currency exchange. I've been there 10 times since hurricane Maria and I keep finding new places to explore during each visit.

Whats is the most important items you have in your carryon and why?

The most important thing in my carry on is probably my spare phone charger and extra bars of soap. My passport or ID is probably the most important things but they're usually not in my carry on.

Favorite Calming Beverage or Food to consume while traveling and why?

I try to drink plenty of water while traveling because I'm always concerned about dehydration. I also like fresh juice. I'll eat almost anything while traveling.

Favorite Calming Music or Audio to listen to while traveling?

I listen to a lot of gospel music.

Favorite Keepsake that keeps you calm or grounded while traveling?

I don't have a favorite keepsake. I travel as light as possible.

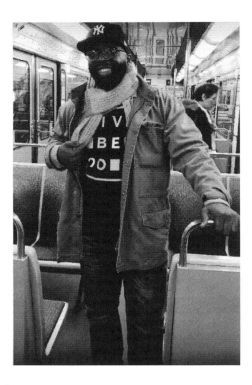

What is your most hilarious travel memory?

> Being drunk in San Juan with 2 childhood friends last October. I can't talk about it and the pictures were destroyed lolol

What is your most memorable or touching travel experience?

> Haiti had a huge impact on me. I cried when it was time to leave. It gave me a new perspective on the quality of life.

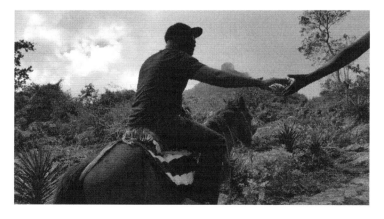

What is the worst travel experience you ever had?

> I haven't had a bad experience yet.

Favorite Travel Hack?

> Google flights

What is your travel Ritual for keeping calm and maintaining your inner zen?

> Pack light. The stress from packing can be enough to make a person second guess whether the trip is even worth it.

Best Travel Tip Advice?

> Just book it!!!

Why is addressing mental health in and self-care with as it relates to people of color so important in the travel community?

> We don't discuss it enough. We don't feel like we have safe places to vent, decompress and disconnect from sources of stress and strife. I believe that more of us are seeing the value of self-care and becoming intentional about protecting our mental health.

Although we travel often for our mental health, the topic is not emphasized due to shame and stigma. How can we normalize this conversation among the travel communities of color?

> People will identify and connect with others who share experiences that resonate with them. The people I interact with regularly are familiar with the term "mental health break". It is a form of medicine for the mind. I think we need to discuss long term benefits of making travel a regular part of our regular routine and lifestyle.

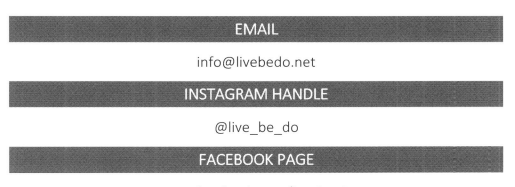

EMAIL
info@livebedo.net

INSTAGRAM HANDLE
@live_be_do

FACEBOOK PAGE
www.facebook.com/live.be.do

Travel Jokes

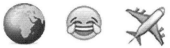

Me trying to explain my itinerary

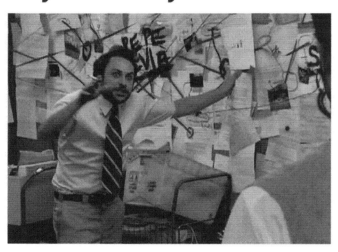

CHAPTER 16

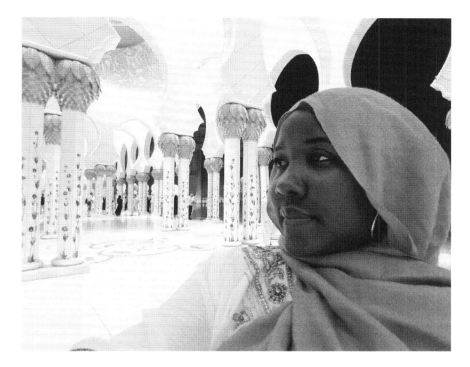

Nubia Young

Women of Color

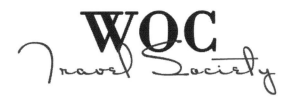

Travel Quote or Travel Mantra you live by
Educate | Empower | Explore

Travel Influencer/ Brand Summary

Created to inspire women of color to be empowered to travel solo and connect with other like-minded female travelers.

How has Traveling helped you maintain your mental health as it relates to self-care?

Traveling has helped me in my pursuit of happiness. It has helped me take my mind off of stressful situations.

What is your most therapeutic travel destination for stress relief and self-care?

Northern Thailand

Whats is the most important items you have in your carryon and why?

Antibacterial wipes, snacks, noise cancelation headphones, warm socks, and a sweater. These are my essentials in my carry on. You do not want to get sick before your adventure even begins and airports and airplanes are full of germs! Wipe down the handles on your seat and your tray table before placing any items or food on it. Snacks are a no brainer! Don't rely on picking something up on your way. Pack snacks in advance. The air conditioning in many places can be on full blast. Having a nice warm pair of socks or a sweater can keep you from being cold and uncomfortable.

Favorite Calming Beverage or Food to consume while traveling and why?

Anything with cucumber or lime! I love a gin and tonic with lime or cucumber water. Popcorn is my go-to food and puts me in a happy space.

Favorite Calming Music or Audio to listen to while traveling?

I listen to Wayne Dyer; Change Your Life, Change Your Mind on Audible

Favorite Keepsake that keeps you calm or grounded while traveling?

Unfortunately, I can't say that I have a favorite keepsake that I travel with.

What is your most hilarious travel memory?

Hmmm, I can't think of one specific moment. I've had so many wonderful experiences. However, I can say that my most memorable experiences are when I make connections with locals or other travelers while traveling. It brings a whole other level to traveling solo.

What is your most memorable or touching travel experience?

One of the most touching experiences was with a young Thai girl in the Southern region of Thailand. I was taking in the sights at a well-known crystal lake in Krabi. The Thai and Chinese people were having a field day, snapping shots of me as I walked by. It was a hot day, so I stopped at one of the stands to purchase a bottle of water. A young girl, no older than 12 years old, stands beside me and begins grinning. She had braces with bright pink rubber bands. I gave her a smile and said Sawadee Kaa (Hello in Thai). Her entire face lit up! She says "Oh, you know Thai", I respond "a little". She then touches my arm and says, "I love your skin. It is so beautiful." I think at that moment, I almost shed a tear. I gave her a hug, told her she was very beautiful herself. It was a touching moment in my travel experience.

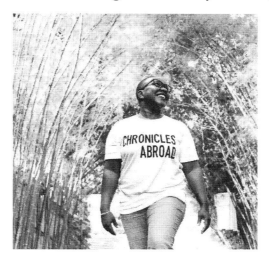

What is the worst travel experience you ever had?

I would have to say India was my worst travel experience. Even as an avid traveler, I did not do the proper research. My experience as a dark skin woman was unpleasant. India views beauty by the color of your skin

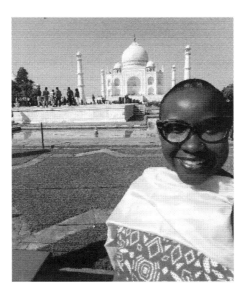

Favorite Travel Hack?

Pack a "get right kit" for a quick freshen-up. Complete with a toothbrush, baby wipes, essential oil or sample size perfume, lotion and deodorant.

What is your travel Ritual for keeping calm and maintaining your inner zen?

Honestly, when I need to recharge. I take a day to do absolutely nothing. No work, no company, no plans. I lay in bed and reflect on my life.

Best Travel Tip Advice?

Do your research about the country before booking flights there. Join a Facebook group specifically about that country or ask someone who has been there. These steps can save you lots of time, money and energy when you are informed and aware.

Why is addressing mental health in and self-care with as it relates to people of color so important in the travel community?

People of color who are avid travelers and ex-pats have the power to share their experiences and educate people on a country or location. Knowledge is power.

Although we travel often for our mental health, the topic is not emphasized due to shame and stigma. How can we normalize this conversation among the travel communities of color?

We need to talk about it! Speak up and voice your experiences with full transparency. No one can shame you if you take back the power of YOUR story and control the narrative!

WEBSITE

www.woctravelsociety.com

EMAIL

nytravelstheworld@gmail.com

INSTAGRAM HANDLE

@anuexperience

FACEBOOK PAGE

WOC Travel Society

Travel Jokes

You've never felt true fear until your passport isn't where you think you left it.

CHAPTER 17

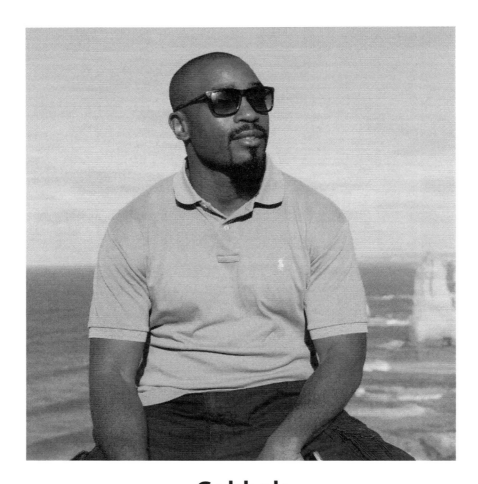

Gabbok

Daddy Day Care Travel Edition

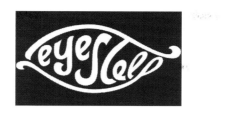

Travel Quote or Travel Mantra you live by
I travel because I don't know enough

How has Traveling helped you maintain your mental health as it relates to self-care?

To be honest, I haven't used travel as self-care. I used to travel to escape the war But I understand the need to breathe in a different environment to recenter ourselves.

What is your most therapeutic travel destination for stress relief and self-care?

Because I travel Around 10 to 15 countries a year. My stress relief is wherever my daughter is.

Whats is the most important items you have in your carryon and why?

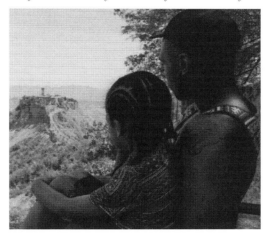

My cameras are my work tools, can't go anywhere without it. I can't afford to capture a moment

Favorite Calming Beverage or Food to consume while traveling and why?

I drink a lot of Redbull, because it keeps me up. And water because it calms me down.

Favorite Calming Music or Audio to listen to while traveling?

I listen to calm electronic music like Petit

Favorite Keepsake that keeps you calm or grounded while traveling?

My two rings: One represents Islam the other one a compass

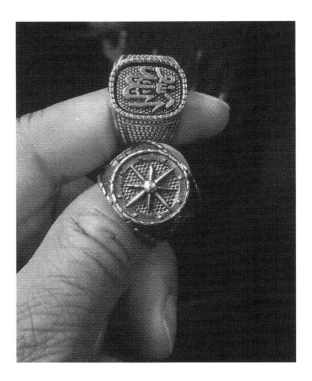

What is your most hilarious travel memory?

I guess traveling my daughter makes my travel with hilarious just by being a father

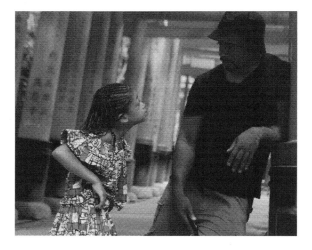

What is your most memorable or touching travel experience?

bring my mother to Asia

What is the worst travel experience you ever had?

Being locked up in jail over seas

Favorite Travel Hack?

Find someone else to pay for it. Incorporate it into your business or find a business other passions. I don't pay my travel

Gabbok

What is your travel Ritual for keeping calm and maintaining your inner zen?

Muslim Prayers

Best Travel Tip Advice?

no plan is the best plan

Why is addressing mental health in and self-care with as it relates to people of color so important in the travel community?

Traveling can be stressful at times. Being a Traveler of color or of a different race or nationality or of different religious practices can be even more stressful. We overlook the importance of self care because we've been taught to remain and stay strong for so long

Although we travel often for our mental health, the topic is not emphasized due to shame and stigma. How can we normalize this conversation among the travel communities of color?

By just talking about it and normalizing the conversation

WEBSITE

www.eyestell.com

EMAIL

gabbok@eyestell.com

INSTAGRAM HANDLE

Gabbok

FACEBOOK PAGE

Gabbok

Travel Jokes

  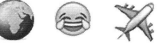

Flewed Out
/flüd out/
verb
When all flight and travel expenses are paid for, "without ones money."

CHAPTER 18

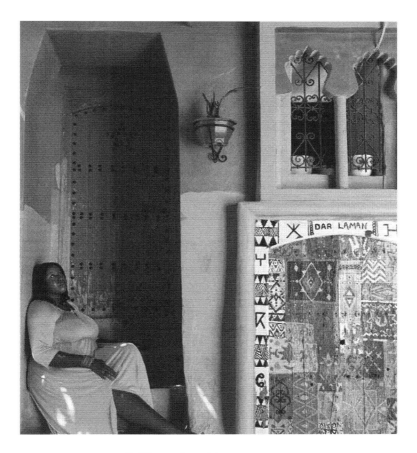

Nicole Brewer
The Globe Trotting Teacher

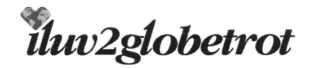

Travel Quote or Travel Mantra you live by
"We travel not to escape life, but for life not to escape us."

Travel Influencer / Brand Summary

I Luv 2 Globe Trot is a travel brand for those interested in traveling and living abroad. Our focus is to inspire others to see the world.

How has Traveling helped you maintain your mental health as it relates to self-care?

I live abroad in a small town called Nizwa in Oman. Traveling is an important part of my self-care in order to keep my sanity since I'm a big city girl living in an unconventional setting.

What is your most therapeutic travel destination for stress relief and self-care?

Zanzibar, Tanzania.

Whats is the most important items you have in your carryon and why?

Small roll-on lavender oil.

Favorite Calming Beverage or Food to consume while traveling and why?

Favorite Calming Music or Audio to listen to while traveling

smooth jazz

Favorite Keepsake that keeps you calm or grounded while traveling?

rose quartz necklace

What is your most hilarious travel memory?

One of my favorite funny travel memories is when I was in India and had to use the bathroom after riding a camel. We were far out from everything and stopped at a little outhouse where a family let me use their "restroom" which was just a little hole in the ground surrounded by a tiny shack. The elderly lady was so amused by my orange nails that her face was priceless while admiring them.

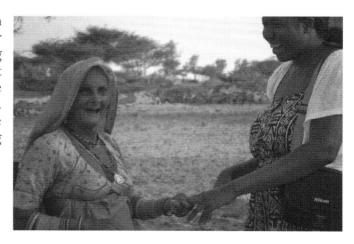

Nicole Brewer

What is your most memorable or touching travel experience?

> One of my most memorable or touching experiences would be when I went on a volunteer trip to Kenya and met the kids at an orphanage in the Kibera slums area.

What is the worst travel experience you ever had?

> One of my worst travel experiences was traveling to Thailand full moon party solo and not being able to access my money due to my card being blocked. It was scary and horrific trying to call a family member or friend in a foreign country with no access to money.

Favorite Travel Hack?

> NA

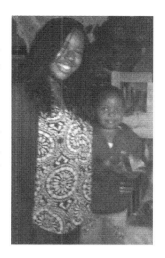

What is your travel Ritual for keeping calm and maintaining your inner zen?

> Prayer

Best Travel Tip Advice?

> Just do it. Don't wait on others to go, live in the moment, travel solo and find yourself. Also, use travel communities like iluv2globetrot for inspiration and travel tips.

Why is addressing mental health in and self-care with as it relates to people of color so important in the travel community?

> Addressing self-care is important for people of color in the travel community because it's imperative to combat the stigma that minorities do not discuss self-care. I feel that people often travel to "get away from it all." Nevertheless, it's important to have a discussion on practical ways to heal during our travels as well.

Although we travel often for our mental health, the topic is not emphasized due to shame and stigma. How can we normalize this conversation among the travel communities of color?

> I think using our travel groups and communities is a start to keep the conversation going about mental health and travel.

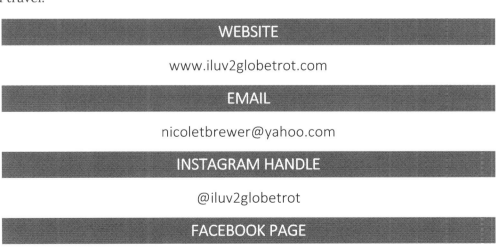

WEBSITE
www.iluv2globetrot.com

EMAIL
nicoletbrewer@yahoo.com

INSTAGRAM HANDLE
@iluv2globetrot

FACEBOOK PAGE
www.facebook.com/iluv2globetro

Travel Jokes

> Don't let a man with NO PASSPORT, tell you that you're the most beautiful girl in the world. How he know sis? He ain't been nowhere 😂😂😂😂😂

CHAPTER 19

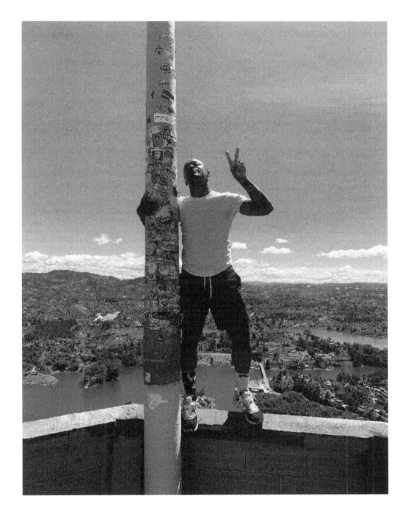

Darnell Walker
The Secret Traveler

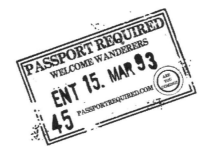

Travel Quote or Travel Mantra you live by
Leave yourself behind.

How has Traveling helped you maintain your mental health as it relates to self-care?

Connecting with other humans and hearing their stories and sharing mine allows me space to be vulnerable and compassionate.

What is your most therapeutic travel destination for stress relief and self-care?

Entrelacs, Quebec

Whats is the most important items you have in your carryon and why?

My Journal!!!

Favorite Calming Beverage or Food to consume while traveling and why?

Absolutely any food without pork. Baby Goat sweetbreads have been the greatest thus far.

Favorite Calming Music or Audio to listen to while traveling?

I have a playlist on Spotify: When Writing or Drinking Whisky

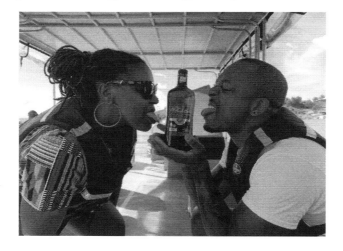

Favorite Keepsake that keeps you calm or grounded while traveling?

Just my journal.

Darnell Walker

What is your most hilarious travel memory?

We were running for the train in France and one of my travelers jumped on ahead of us all and the doors shut. It was her first time out of the county and watching her face as the train pulled off was hilarious and also frightening. She lived and laughed.

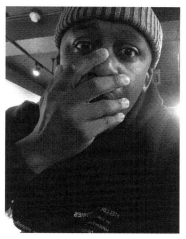

What is your most memorable or touching travel experience?

Doing shrooms in an open field in Quebec while watching the stars with some of the most amazing people I know.

What is the worst travel experience you ever had?

I had an awful person traveling with me who was absolutely negative about everything. She brought the energy down around her.

Favorite Travel Hack?

Asking for a wheelchair at the ticket counter when you're late for your flight and the security line is long.

What is your travel Ritual for keeping calm and maintaining your inner zen?

I write!

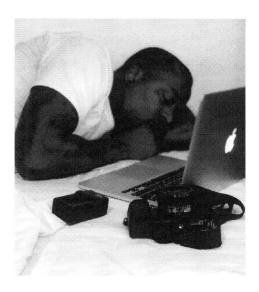

The Ultimate Self-Care Guide for Travelers of Color

Best Travel Tip Advice?

Leave everyone behind and go!

Why is addressing mental health in and self-care with as it relates to people of color so important in the travel community?

Look ain't nobody gonna help us! We have to help ourselves and each other. There are way too many stories of us dying from suicide.

Although we travel often for our mental health, the topic is not emphasized due to shame and stigma. How can we normalize this conversation among the travel communities of color?

Behind each Traveler is a story about mental health. We gotta share our stories often to help others. One of the many reasons I created the "Outside The House " a documentary about mental health and people courageously sharing their stories breaking cycles that are killing us in dark places.

WEBSITE

Passportrequired.com

EMAIL

darnell.walker@me.com

INSTAGRAM HANDLE

PassportReq

FACEBOOK PAGE

PassportRequired

WEBSITE

Passportrequired.com

Travel Jokes

 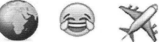

When Big Sean said, "f**k a vacay, I feel better at work" .... I never sing that part. 🙅

CHAPTER 20

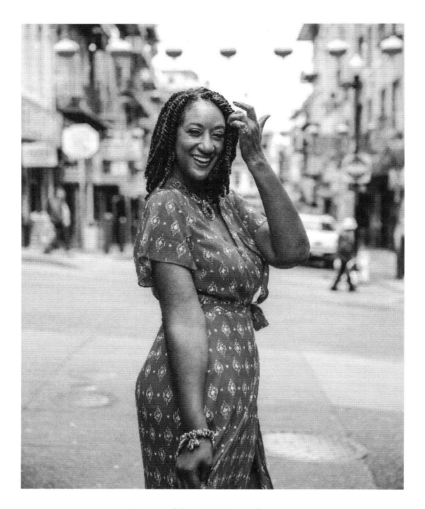

Sonjia Mackey

Beast Mode

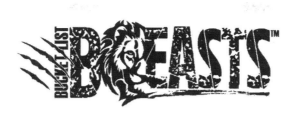

Travel Quote or Travel Mantra you live by
I'm not afraid of death. I'm afraid of being alive and not living.

Travel Influencer/ Brand Summary

"Bucket List Beasts" is a travel, adventure, and life inspiration company created to help people design and live purpose-driven, passion-filled lives full of fun, freedom, and fulfillment. The Founder, Mediocrity Escapologist Sonjia "Lioness" Mackey, has traveled to all 50 states and more than 79 different countries across all 7 continents while passionately and relentlessly checking destinations and adventures off her beloved bucket list

How has Traveling helped you maintain your mental health as it relates to self-care?

For many years, I used travel as a form of mental, physical, and emotional escape. If I wasn't actually on a trip, I was planning one or dreaming about one. No matter what was going on in my life, just having a trip booked seemed to make everything better. Now, I've created a life I don't need to escape from. And that's because my business and lifestyle are rooted in my favorite form of self-care – travel. I'm 100% location-independent which allows me to live a life of travel continuously, not just as a form of periodic escapism.

What is your most therapeutic travel destination for stress relief and self-care?

The wilds of Africa, where I can experience natural occurrences vs. "man-made" ones.

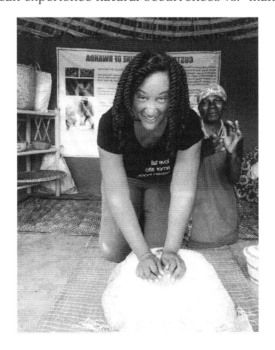

Whats is the most important items you have in your carryon and why?

Laptop, tablet, or phone. I'm a busy entrepreneur trying to build an empire. Additionally, I'm always thinking of new business ideas and there are several books I want to write. Honestly, I could live three lifetimes and probably not accomplish everything I want to do. The beauty of it all is that my business is rooted in my purpose and passions. I get to serve others and make a difference in the world using my gifts, skills, and talents to do work I love, from anywhere in the world!

Favorite Calming Beverage or Food to consume while traveling and why?

I'm a "Junk Food Junkie" and I make no apologies for it! That means I always have sweet and salty snacks on hand. Some of my favorites: Reese's Peanut Butter Cups, Lay's Potato Chips, Peanut M&M's, and Mr. Goodbar. I'm also a connoisseur of cheeseburgers and fries and try to partake in the best local offerings wherever I go.

Favorite Calming Music or Audio to listen to while traveling?

I'm not a huge music listener while traveling. Instead, I'm a big movie-watcher. So I always have movies downloaded on my phone, tablet, or laptop. However, on the occasions when I do prefer music to relax, classic rock and R&B from the 70's, 80's, and 90's are my go-to selections.

Favorite Keepsake that keeps you calm or grounded while traveling?

I don't have one. I'm nomadic by nature. I was born to be a wanderer. I'm like the song, "Papa Was a Rolling Stone" and the verse, "Wherever he laid his hat was his home." Wherever I lay my purse and set down my luggage is my home. Home is wherever I am, even if it's just for a moment in time. That nomadic, wandering mentality, oddly enough, calms and grounds me.

What is your most hilarious travel memory?

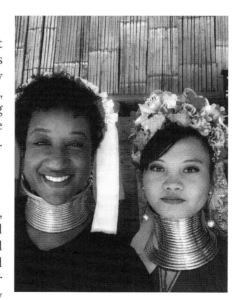

My first trip to Thailand. It was like the movie "Hangover" – only it was happening to me! It was a series of mishaps and misadventures that I could only laugh about, even as they were happening. Like how I asked the taxi driver to take me to a ping-pong show, as in the sport, and he took me to a ping-pong show, as in nude people performing sexual acts! I remember thinking to myself, "At what point did we [the taxi driver and I] have a breakdown in communication?" LOL. For the record, I stayed until the end of the show though! LOL.

What is your most memorable or touching travel experience?

The first time I went to Africa in 2005, I went to Kenya and Tanzania, specifically, places like the Masai Mara, the Serengeti, and Ngorongoro Crater. These were places I grew up watching and hearing about as a child via shows like Discovery Channel and National Geographic. I told myself, "I'm going to see those places for myself someday." So in 2005, I literally had tears rolling down my cheeks as I stood on the deck of my glamping tent looking out across the Serengeti, thanking God because I made it. I made it!

What is the worst travel experience you ever had?

Honestly, I can't say that I've had a "worst" travel experience. Obviously, there are destinations I've been disappointed in (typically in Europe because some countries lack the level of adventure I prefer). But I've always felt that every country has advantages and disadvantages and I go in determined to find those advantages – the best that a particular country has to offer. Travel is what we make of it. It's often about what we bring to a destination, not what a destination has to offer us. If you adopt the right mindset and set your expectations going in, you can make the best out of any "worst" travel experience.

Favorite Travel Hack?

Anything that allows me to travel more and/or do it less expensively, or better yet, for free. So that would be credit card and frequent traveler program hacking.

What is your travel Ritual for keeping calm and maintaining your inner zen?

I'm a "Spa Baby" and "Bath Junkie" – so I'm always on the look-out for an unusual bathtub (in terms of shape, location, view, etc.) or unique spa treatment during my travels. Some of the more unusual spa treatments I've had: a live snake massage, a bird-poop facial, a bamboo stick massage, a butt facial, a massage by a blind person, and much more!

Best Travel Tip Advice?

There are so many misconceptions about travel, most of which are rooted in fear. Fear is the #1 thing keeping most people from pursuing their dreams and living their lives to the fullest. You have one life. Just one. So why aren't you running like you're on fire toward your wildest dreams? Don't wait until it's time to die to find out you never really lived. Just do it. Because you don't overcome fear by not doing what scares you; you overcome fear by doing the very thing that scares you!

Why is addressing mental health in and self-care with as it relates to people of color so important in the travel community?

Mental health has a history of being a taboo topic amongst people of color. It's not a topic we acknowledge or openly discuss. But not talking about something or acting as if it doesn't exist doesn't make it go away. It just makes it more difficult for the people who need help to admit they need help and then to get the help they need. And let's keep it real – if there's one thing about those tables, they always Honestly, I can't say that I've had a "worst" travel experience. Obviously, there are destinations I've been disappointed in (typically in Europe because some countries lack the level of adventure I prefer). But I've always felt that every country has advantages and disadvantages and I go in determined to find those advantages – the best that a particular country has to offer. Travel is what we make of it. It's often about what we bring to a destination, not what a destination has to offer us. If you adopt the right mindset and set your expectations going in, you can make the best out of any "worst" travel experience.

Anything that allows me to travel more and/or do it less expensively, or better yet, for free. So that would be credit card and frequent traveler program hacking.?

I'm a "Spa Baby" and "Bath Junkie" – so I'm always on the look-out for an unusual bathtub (in terms of shape, location, view, etc.) or unique spa treatment during my travels. Some of the more unusual spa treatments I've had: a live snake massage, a bird-poop facial, a bamboo stick massage, a butt facial, a massage by a blind person, and much more!

There are so many misconceptions about travel, most of which are rooted in fear. Fear is the #1 thing keeping most people from pursuing their dreams and living their lives to the fullest. You have one life. Just one. So why aren't you running like you're on fire toward your wildest dreams? Don't wait until it's time to die to find out you never really lived. Just do it. Because you don't overcome fear by not doing what scares you; you overcome fear by doing the very thing that scares you!

Mental health has a history of being a taboo topic amongst people of color. It's not a topic we acknowledge or openly discuss. But not talking about something or acting as if it doesn't exist doesn't make it go away.

It just makes it more difficult for the people who need help to admit they need help and then to get the help they need. And let's keep it real – if there's one thing about those tables

Never know when we will find our own selves in the position of needing to discuss or get help for our own mental health concerns.?

Turn. Meaning we never know when we will find our own selves in the position of needing to discuss or get help for our own mental health concerns.

Although we travel often for our mental health, the topic is not emphasized due to shame and stigma. How can we normalize this conversation among the travel communities of color?

Frankly, just opening the door to more discussion about mental health is a way to help normalize it. It's like racism. The conversations may get ugly, and things may get said in the hurt or anger of the moment, but getting things out in the open is the only chance we have at confronting the issue head-on, thereby increasing awareness and bringing the topic out of the dark and into the light so people can get the help they need. We can't change what we're not willing to face.

WEBSITE

www.sonjiamackey.com

EMAIL

sonjia@bucketlistbeasts.com

INSTAGRAM HANDLE

@BucketListBeasts

FACEBOOK PAGE

https://www.facebook.com/groups/BucketListBeasts/

Travel Jokes

If he isn't down to travel, gotta let that

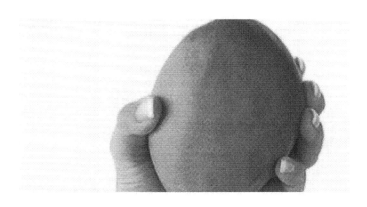

CHAPTER 21

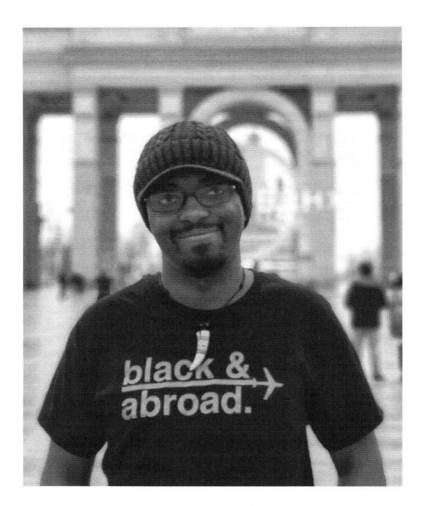

Leroy Tyler

A Black Man Abroad

A BLACK MAN ABROAD

Travel Quote or Travel Mantra you live by
Everything you've ever wanted is on the other side of fear

How has Traveling helped you maintain your mental health as it relates to self-care?

It allows me to discover more about who I am as a person, what I can/can't handle, and who I can/can't trust.

What is your most therapeutic travel destination for stress relief and self-care?

Fiji. The ocean, the beautiful sunsets, and the people make Fiji a perfect destination to relieve stress

Whats is the most important items you have in your carryon and why?

A pen to fill out the immigration form, my neck pillow, gum, and snacks to eat in between meals on long flights

Favorite Calming Beverage or Food to consume while traveling and why?

caramel Frappuccino with extra caramel

Favorite Calming Music or Audio to listen to while traveling?

Ambient trance

Favorite Keepsake that keeps you calm or grounded while traveling?

My mother's obituary. That way, she's with me everywhere I go

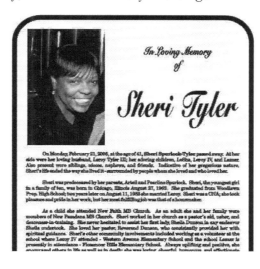

What is your most hilarious travel memory?

When I went to Russia this past March. I was able to wear a big fur coat and a ushanka while in an ice bar. I sampled some vodka and caviar. It was the most disgusting thing ever. My facial expressions were priceless

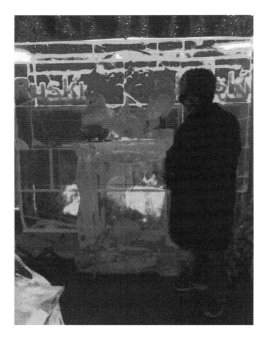

What is your most memorable or touching travel experience?

Visiting Chernobyl. I've read about it and watched dozens of documentaries on it. Seeing it for myself is by far the coolest thing I've ever done

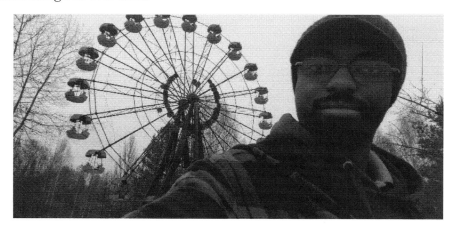

Favorite Travel Hack?

If you live in, or near Chi ago, and if you need a passport in a hurry, you can go to the Dirkson Federal Building downtown with proof of travel within 14 days, and all necessary documents, you'll receive your passport within 6 hours

What is your travel Ritual for keeping calm and maintaining your inner zen?

If something happens, I tell myself it could be a lot worse

Best Travel Tip Advice?

Be flexible with your travel dates. Pushing your travel dates out by 1 day can decrease the price significantly

Why is addressing mental health in and self-care with as it relates to people of color so important in the travel community?

Addressing mental health/self-care is so important to people of color because it's often stigmatized. There was this toxic, generational mindset of "Whatever happens in this house, stays in this house ", making it difficult to open up. Travel has really help me cope with it. It's allowed me to be more adventurous, well rounded, and to be temporarily freed from any negativity brewing in my brain.

Although we travel often for our mental health, the topic is not emphasized due to shame and stigma. How can we normalize this conversation among the travel communities of color?

We can normalize the conversation by traveling with like minded people, and speak to them about their coping mechanisms while they travel, and compare and contrast. It creates an awesome networking opportunity as well

WEBSITE
Ablackmanabroad.com

EMAIL
bruceleroy36@gmail.com

INSTAGRAM HANDLE
@ablackmanabroad

FACEBOOK PAGE
https://m.facebook.com/leroy.tyleriv.3?ref=bookmarks

Travel Jokes

first date idea: the airport. if they're incompetent and slow in the security line you can just cut it off then and there

CHAPTER 22

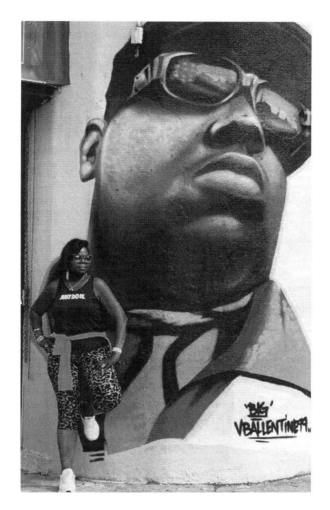

Eartha Franklin

That WoW Factor !

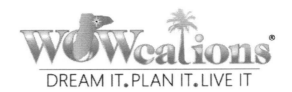

Travel Quote or Travel Mantra you live by

That moment you realize life isn't about having it all.
It's about creating, cultivating and sharing experiences
that define your true essence, unapologetically.

Travel Influencer / Brand Summary

WOWCATIONS was started to put the WOWfactor in traveling. We ensure that your travel experience is one to remember! Whether you're planning a family vacation, group vacation, Baecation, mental retreat or just want a short get-a-way, we ensure that you return home with memories to boast about. We offer full-service travel arrangements including airport transportation, transfers at your destination, travel insurance to protect your trip and guided tours. It's our obligation to ensure your vacation is a WOWcation!

How has Traveling helped you maintain your mental health as it relates to self-care?

Travel has helped me tremendously in my day to day life. Planning and waiting for each trip to come keeps my mind focused on the destinations I've chosen and away from all the stress that I deal with on a daily basis. I am always thinking about my next adventure!

What is your most therapeutic travel destination for stress relief and self-care?

Bali, Indonesia afforded me the opportunity to unwind, let my hair down, and get pampered while being a kid again. I am able to laugh while I'm there, rise with the sun, pray with the Gods and soak in the finest baths known to man. Bali man, yea, I really dig it.

Whats is the most important items you have in your carryon and why?

My phone & charger! The combo ensures that I was able to capture a minute of my travel experiences so I can share them with my family & followers.

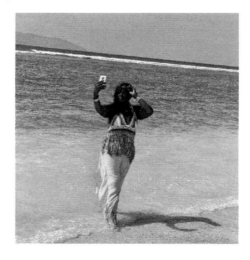

Eartha Franklin

Favorite Calming Beverage or Food to consume while traveling and why?

    Any well mixed alcoholic beverage makes me feel relaxed and all grown up during my travels

Favorite Calming Music or Audio to listen to while traveling?

    Neo Soul & Good Jazz

Favorite Keepsake that keeps you calm or grounded while traveling?

    My 5 grandsons. I always look forward to creating memories & stories to share with them. I also ensure I make safe decisions along my travels so I make it home to them.

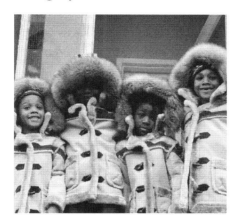
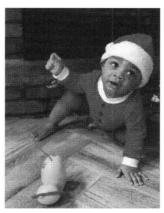

What is your most hilarious travel memory?

    Climbing my fat azz up on the camel in Egypt! It took my husband and 5 other people to convince me to get on the camel and when I did, the camel raised his back legs uplifting me off the ground and I thought I would die! I screamed so loud even the pyramids heard me!

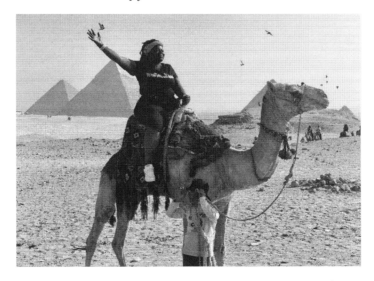

Am O'Dell I, Kenya, East Africa when the Masai tribe surprisingly greeted us in their traditional chant & prayer welcoming us to the motherland! I also got to spend time with the children of the tribe. I will never forget that day! I cried. My husband cried. We all cried.

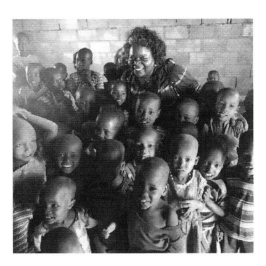

Favorite Travel Hack?

- Most of my trips are flights that require me to be in the air for longer than 10 hours. Here's how I handle long flights:
- I usually book early morning flights so I do not sleep the night before.
- I make a run to the liquor store and purchase 5 nip bottles of my fav alcohol I clean my house, throw out the garbage, empty the fridge from leftovers, pay bills, die load movies to my phone, check my packing and repack if necessary, etc.
- On the morning of the flight, I eat a good breakfast prior to leaving the house.
- I uber it to the airport consuming one of the nips on the way
- Once I check-in and clear customs, I consume 2 more nips [theyre 1oz bottles so they're allowed past customs]

By the time I board my flight I'm nice & lit. I may hit one more bottle but so can assure you that by the time the flight leaves the tarmac I am out cold and will sleep for hours. By the time I wake up I'm usually halfway or close to my destination.

What is your travel Ritual for keeping calm and maintaining your inner zen?

Don't sweat the small stuff. Embrace the cultural differences along my journey, it's what makes the destination enlightening and interesting. Take deep breaths of the country's fresh air. Leave a sprinkle of you everywhere you go!

Best Travel Tip Advice?

Book early. Use credit cards that give great travel rewards. Don't be afraid to travel where your friends dare to go.

Why is addressing mental health in and self-care with as it relates to people of color so important in the travel community?

Because it's the 5,000-pound elephant in the room. We all know it's there but few from the black and brown travel community talk about it and how it's impacting our relationships, friendships, families and communities. Sharing our feelings and emotions is not only healthy, it also helps the person you're sharing with who may be afraid of opening up due to being judged or looked down upon. We're all going through something. Finding opportunities to share, connect and divulge is cleansing

Eartha Franklin

Although we travel often for our mental health, the topic is not emphasized due to shame and stigma. How can we normalize this conversation among the travel communities of color?

Open forums, Whiteboards, Social media groups, breakout sessions during major travel events. Any place where we are free to discuss without reproach.

WEBSITE

www.mywowcations.com

EMAIL

travelbyeartha@gmail.com

INSTAGRAM HANDLE

https://www.instagram.com/mywowcations

FACEBOOK PAGE

https://www.instagram.com/mywowcations

Travel Jokes

MY HEART

Looking at travel blogs	
Researching my next trip	
Hitting book on plane tickets	

CHAPTER 23

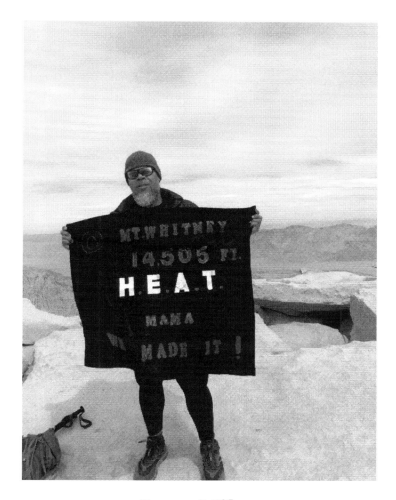

Stan Miles

Bringing the Heat

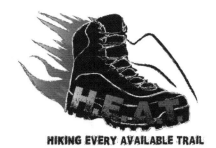

Travel Quote or Travel Mantra you live by
"And into the forest I go, to lose my mind and find my soul".
John Muir

Travel Influencer/ Brand Summary
> Hiking Trail group that travels all over California and beyond.

How has Traveling helped you maintain your mental health as it relates to self-care?
> Most of my traveling involves being outdoors the majority of the time. Being close to nature with good people and beautiful sights allows me to forget the worries of the world that I may carry at any particular time. Fresh air and the sense of accomplishment during hikes are euphoric.

What is your most therapeutic travel destination for stress relief and self-care?
> Yosemite National Park. It's a 3-hour drive for me which is therapeutic in itself. Being amongst the waterfalls and huge slabs of granite is like the Disneyland for hikers.

Whats is the most important items you have in your carryon and why?
> My mini speaker. Music and exercise go hand in hand with me.

Favorite Calming Beverage or Food to consume while traveling and why?
> Summit victory peanut M&M's. Reaching my destination is that much more enjoyable when I know I have my M&M reward.

Favorite Calming Music or Audio to listen to while traveling?
> I have a hiking playlist that consists of rap, r&b, and oldies mostly that I play every hike.

Favorite Keepsake that keeps you calm or grounded while traveling?
> Nothing in particular

What is your most hilarious travel memory?
> Making it to the top of the highest peak in the contiguous United States and proposing to the mountain.

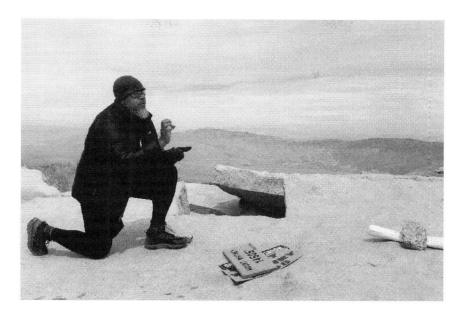

What is your most memorable or touching travel experience?

> Taking about 60 people to Zion National Park last year, most of them, people of color. In Utah, that's a huge thing to introduce us to different paths of the outdoors.

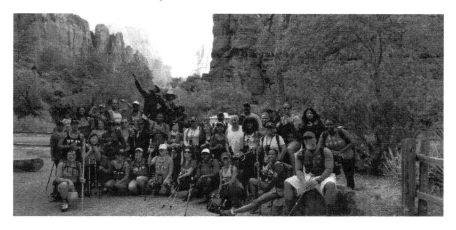

What is the worst travel experience you ever had?

> Not sure if I've had one. When you are in your element, you can make the best out of situations that aren't always ideal.

Favorite Travel Hack?

What is your travel Ritual for keeping calm and maintaining your inner zen?

> Maintaining patience. My travel usually involves a number of people which means multiple personalities. Patience is something needed and transferred to everyday life as well.

Best Travel Tip Advice?

> Explore more but don't limit yourself to only what's seen on social media. Great trips can be a 15-hour plane ride or a few hours in the car. Open-minded traveling keeps the stress levels down and the happiness elevated.

Why is addressing mental health in and self-care with as it relates to people of color so important in the travel community?

There are so many stereotypes regarding POC and our travel habits. It's not a normal occurrence to see us or hear about us in travel circles. Although it's slowly changing, there's still a ways to go before the reasoning is mainstream in our conversations. Everyone needs an outlet, and hiking/traveling is mine. My body and mental thanks me every hike.

Although we travel often for our mental health, the topic is not emphasized due to shame and stigma. How can we normalize this conversation among the travel communities of color?

By simply starting the conversation and inviting others to join in. Like what you're doing basically. I often get plenty of members to tell me they need(Ed) our weekly hike after the week they've had for their mental health. As we get older, I believe we're less likely to shame the conversation and more likely to contribute and share experiences with others.

WEBSITE

HeatHikes.com

EMAIL

heathikes@gmail.com

INSTAGRAM HANDLE

Stan Miles

Travel Jokes

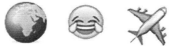

Day 147 without sex: I went through the airport metal detector with a fork in my pocket just so someone could feel me up.

CHAPTER 24

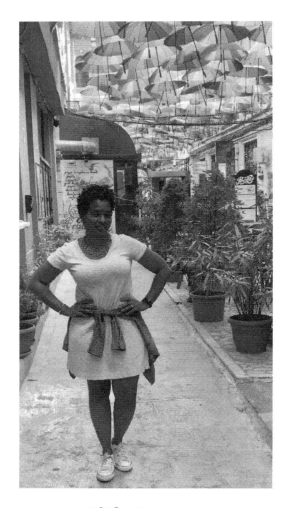

Jill Carter

Fly Mommy

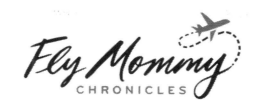

Travel Quote or Travel Mantra you live by
Collect memories, not things!

Travel Influencer/ Brand Summary

Fly Mommy Chronicles is a brand committed to inspiring moms of color to travel and see the world! Whether it's with family, significant other, friends or solo....I encourage Fly Mommies to get out there and #booktheflight! Traveling is an amazing source of self-care for busy moms who are pulled and stretched in a million directions.

How has Traveling helped you maintain your mental health as it relates to self-care?

It helps with the mommy blues that can sometimes be overwhelming. It provides a balance. It recharges me mentally and spiritually so that I am healthy.

What is your most therapeutic travel destination for stress relief and self-care?

Most people are drawn to beaches for self-care and stress relief. Give me a big city to wander around and sit and people watch and then watch my stress melt away! Paris always comes to mind for this purpose.

Whats is the most important items you have in your carryon and why?

Clorox wipes to clean the surfaces I come into contact with, a good book, a chic travel blanket/scarf and a great lip gloss so that I can feel fabulous when I get to my destination!

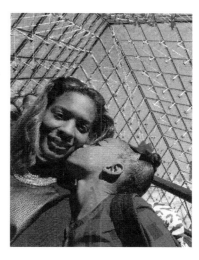

Favorite Calming Beverage or Food to consume while traveling and why?

I love a glass of champagne or rosé to kick off my travels or celebrate the end of a great trip before heading home. This is a great balance between calm and celebratory.

Favorite Calming Music or Audio to listen to while traveling?

Soothing jazz or r&b

Favorite Keepsake that keeps you calm or grounded while traveling?

I always have an actual picture of my family, a new selfie of me and my girls if I'm traveling without them as the new wallpaper on my phone and my travel journal.

What is your most hilarious travel memory?

What is your most memorable or touching travel experience?

> My most memorable travel experience is traveling to Cartagena, Colombia and visiting the town of San Basilio de Palenque. This is the first town of freed slaves in the Americas. It was truly a blessing to visit and learn the history of Palenque through Alex Rocha of Experience Real Cartagena.

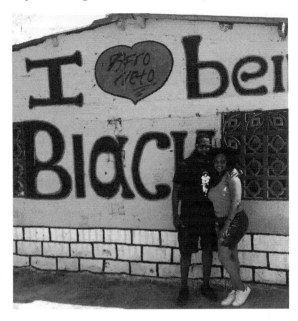

What is the worst travel experience you ever had?

> Getting stuck in Buenos Aires on NYE during our honeymoon. Not the best way to spend your first NYE as a married couple.

Favorite Travel Hack?

> Packing cubes; keeping a scanned copy of my passport in my email; a well-stocked electronics bag with all the cords, battery packs and converters I need.

What is your travel Ritual for keeping calm and maintaining your inner zen?

> I try to stay in a spiritual place when I travel, both thanking God for the opportunity to experience new places and actively seeking Him while I'm away from the grind of my life.

Best Travel Tip Advice?

> Just. Go.

Why is addressing mental health in and self-care with as it relates to people of color so important in the travel community?

> Many of us are suffering in silence. There's nothing wrong with acknowledging that travel is a great way to get a break from stress and come back refreshed and rejuvenated. In fact, that's one of the biggest benefits of travel for me.

Although we travel often for our mental health, the topic is not emphasized due to shame and stigma. How can we normalize this conversation among the travel communities of color?

Jill Carter

We need to keep having the conversation in order to normalize and reduce the stigma. Good mental health...or even lack thereof is real. We can also realize that self-care and mental health are synonymous. Travel is an excellent way to stay on top of both.

WEBSITE

www.flymommychronicles.com

EMAIL

attyjcarter@gmail.com

INSTAGRAM HANDLE

Flymommychronicles

FACEBOOK PAGE

Fly Mommy Chronicles

Travel Jokes

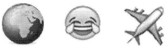

Me: books plane ticket

my bank account:

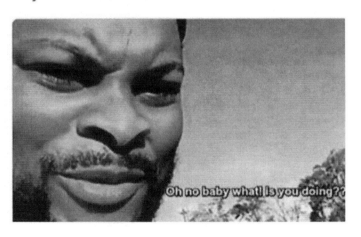

CHAPTER 25

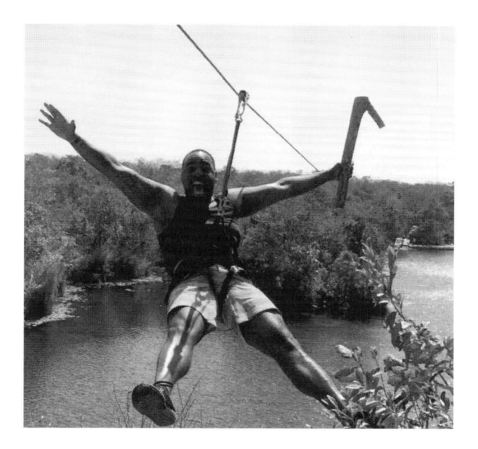

Roland Parker

Black Nomad

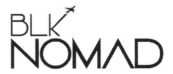

Travel Quote or Travel Mantra you live by
Do not see obstacles, see opportunities.

How has Traveling helped you maintain your mental health as it relates to self-care?

Traveling gives you the opportunity to "reset". It takes you from the everyday wheel of life that can bring us down or drain our energy. Many times you will find clarity by simply thinking in a different space.

What is your most therapeutic travel destination for stress relief and self-care?

Boracay Island is by far my favorite thus far. The white sand beaches alone are enough. However, there are many other amenities; massages, paddleboards, jet skis and even a small nightlife for our dancers.

Whats is the most important items you have in your carryon and why?

Passports. Motrin/pain medicine. Neck pillows. Headphones. Extra shirt/shorts in the event our luggage is lost in transit. Toothbrush/toiletries.

Favorite Calming Beverage or Food to consume while traveling and why?

My new favorite beverage is from the Dominican Republic (probably because we received a cool picture). It is called Mama Juana. I keep the food simple when traveling abroad. Burgers/fries...

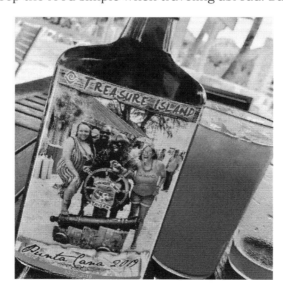

Favorite Calming Music or Audio to listen to while traveling?

I love listening to 90's R&B; very soothing when on a plane as it helps me sleep while in flight.

Favorite Keepsake that keeps you calm or grounded while traveling?

My wife is what keeps me calm when traveling. She is with me 99% of the time.

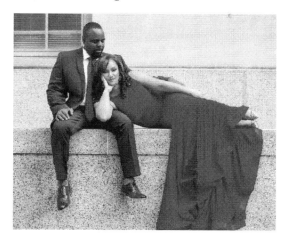

What is your most hilarious travel memory?

My most memorable/hilarious moment was my first-time zip lining. I was so, so nervous and the tour guide pushed me off before being mentally prepared.

What is your most memorable or touching travel experience?

The most touching travel experience was Boracay Island as this was my honeymoon.

What is the worst travel experience you ever had?

The hotel in the Dominican was very unorganized. They kept losing our reservations and the simplest thing; the key to the room kept being deactivated.

Favorite Travel Hack?

When traveling to all-inclusive resorts, bring small bills for tipping. No need to bring 20's as you will be given change in the other country's currency.

What is your travel Ritual for keeping calm and maintaining your inner zen?

My ritual is laying on the beach and finding a place to get a massage. From there, we find all of the water sports possible.

Best Travel Tip Advice?

Respect I love listening to 90's R&B; very soothing when on a plane as it helps me sleep while in flight.

My wife is what keeps me calm when traveling. She is with me 99% of the time.

My most memorable/hilarious moment was my first-time zip lining. I was so, so nervous and the tour guide pushed me off before being mentally prepared.

The most touching travel experience was Boracay Island as this was my honeymoon.

The hotel in the Dominican was very unorganized. They kept losing our reservations and the simplest thing; the key to the room kept being deactivated.

When traveling to all-inclusive resorts, bring small bills for tipping. No need to bring 20's as you will be given change in the other country's currency.

My ritual is laying on the beach and finding a place to get a massage. From there, we find all of the water sports possible.

Best Travel Tip Advice?

Respect others. Respect the culture of where you're visiting. Being kind and respectful will ensure you have a good time and make it home safely.

Why is addressing mental health in and self-care with as it relates to people of color so important in the travel community?

Mental health is almost taboo in the black community. Any mental issues are considered a sign of weakness; therefore most of us will suppress those feelings. This is especially common in black men. We are told to be strong, be emotionless. Awareness is very, very important.

Although we travel often for our mental health, the topic is not emphasized due to shame and stigma. How can we normalize this conversation among the travel communities of color?

By creating an open dialogue. Again, we do not discuss this topic because we do not want to be considered weak. Simply asking, "how are you really doing?" will give someone an opportunity to open up.

WEBSITE

blk-nomad.myshopify.com

EMAIL

rbparker2@gmail.com

INSTAGRAM HANDLE

Blkn0mad

FACEBOOK PAGE

Blck Nomad

Travel Jokes

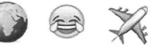

Bae: "Promise me you wont show yo ass on this trip...."

Me: "I promise....."

Me on the trip:

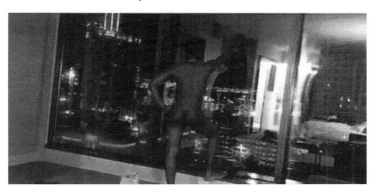

CHAPTER 26

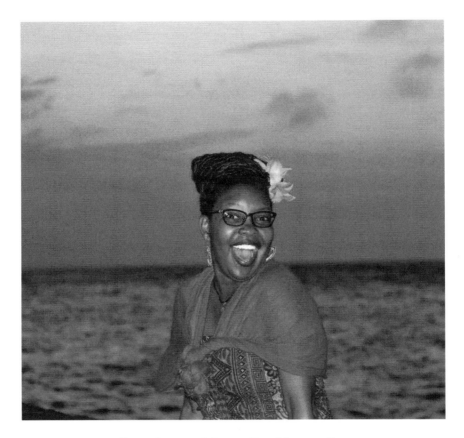

Slyvia (Sly) Callendar

There's Two Sides to This

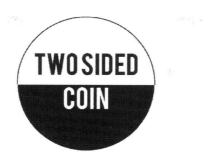

Travel Quote or Travel Mantra you live by
"How long do we have to stare at it?"

Travel Influencer/ Brand Summary

We are an African American couple exploring the world together and documenting our experiences while providing some social commentary. We highlight the challenges of traveling as a couple (internal) while highlighting the unique challenges of traveling while black. We also aim to inspire black love and show that it is possible and does exist. Most recently, we partnered with Knock Out Abuse – West Coast Chapter to promote awareness of domestic abuse and raise money for abuse shelters. For more information and to support, visit; https://twosidedcoin.org/org/.

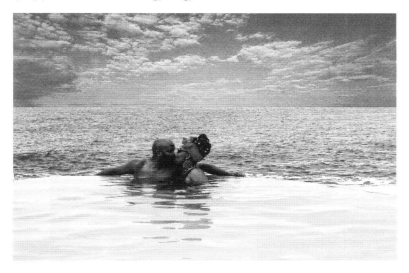

How has Traveling helped you maintain your mental health as it relates to self-care?

Everyday responsibilities can be a grind. Getting up early or working late hours. Fighting traffic, putting up with annoying co-workers or customers, paying bills, the car breaking down just when you don't have a cent to spare, this list is endless. Life is hard. Travel for me is the proverbial silver lining on this cloud of responsibilities and stressors. Knowing that I have an upcoming trip to an exotic place I have never been before being my daily elixir to whatever may come my way. It's like the carrot at the end of the stick; when times are tough, I remind myself that it's not so bad because "I am going to Morroco next month."

What is your most therapeutic travel destination for stress relief and self-care?

Without a doubt, it is Jamaica for me. I am not talking about the famous resorts (which are fantastic, I am sure), but rather the hidden gems, unspoiled by over-tourism where you can disconnect and unwind in utter paradise. I have a few spots that will completely blow your mind. Follow on Instagram

@thetwosidedcoin or subscribe to the blog twosidedcoin.org for a feature article on these (secret) serene secret spots.

Whats is the most important items you have in your carryon and why?

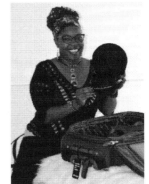

My headphones! I always have my headphones when traveling, for various reasons. Firstly, during the long, stressful airport transitions, nothing calms you down like your favorite sound. Whether its a fave music tune or the reassuring voice of your meditation coach, it is an instant mood lifter. The headphones also ensure that I have a restful, quiet flight. I once sat next to a gentleman who talked to me for 3 hours straight. He ignored all social cues and hints and just went on about himself. Put some headphones on, and everybody leaves you alone.

Favorite Calming Beverage or Food to consume while traveling and why?

Nothing says vacation mode more than a well prepared, fruity cocktail that you can guiltlessly order at noon on a Tuesday! Arguably the most stressful part of Traveling is the airport. So, I have given myself something to look forward to at airports. We get there early and relax with an indulgent fruity drink and relax into vacation mode. It's incredible how this ritual transforms my mindset from Go! Go! Go! To; ok, so the flight has been delayed an hour? I wonder if I have time to try something else. Travel tip: If you travel often, make airports a destination by enrolling in a program that offers access to exclusive airport lounges like Priority Pass®. Disclaimer; The nurse in me has to remind everybody – always drink responsibly.

Favorite Calming Music or Audio to listen to while traveling?

If I had to choose a favorite musician to travel to, it would have to be Cesaria Evora. Her angelic voice accompanied by those exquisite Spanish-style strings are enough to instantly transport you to a beach somewhere, where you are being served a fruity drink by a gorgeous, tall, dark, and handsome bartender named Alessandro. (sigh!) Alessandro!

Favorite Keepsake that keeps you calm or grounded while traveling?

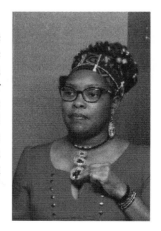

A few years ago, my Mum brought me a chain from Kenya. I wore the chain the first time John and I traveled together. This was the first time I visited somewhere other than Kenya (where I was born). That first trip with John I met his Mum in London, after which, we went to Paris and a few other European cities. I will never forget the feeling I had as I traveled across Europe. This girl from humble beginnings was on a plane bound for Paris! I remember holding the chain and recalling all the hard work and sacrifices that my Mum had had to endure for me to be here. At that moment, the chain took on a significance that has stayed with me ever since. Every time I sit on a plane, I clutch the chain and whisper a thank you to my dear Mother.

What is your most hilarious travel memory?

On our last trip to Europe, we wanted to experience more off-the-beaten-path stuff. So John booked us into a houseboat in Oudendijk. This accommodation was like nothing we had ever done before. The boat was in a small village, isolated from, well, everything. The host built this boat himself and was immensely proud of it, and for a good reason. It was a beautiful, cozy houseboat. John, however, forget to mention that the boat had no plumbing! We would have to shower and do our...ehm, 'paperwork,' outside! The outhouse that doubled as a shower was visible from the canal; we had to be strategic about when to shower; otherwise, the locals would be introduced to a side of us they rather not be. Furthermore, it was a bit of a distance from the outhouse to the boat. During the day, this was not a big deal, but at night, with no light other than moon and stars, it was an adventure to get to. One that I was not brave enough to attempt. So that host kindly provided me with a bucket toilet (a bucket lined with a plastic bag, with some water at the bottom and a sit on the rim) that I could pee in at night without leaving the boat. One night I had to do more than pee. John has never looked at me the same again.

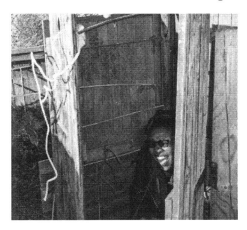

What is your most memorable or touching travel experience?

This award goes to my trip to Cuba. We went to Cuba at a time when Trump had just been elected president and was rolling back a lot of Obama-era policies. These policies included the Cuban embargo Obama had eased during his presidency that allowed Americans to travel to Cuba more easily. We booked the trip a week out; it was a spur of the moment trip. You do not travel to Cuba "spur of the moment"! There are precise stipulations that you have to meet to go to Cuba legally; you can read all about them here; https://twosidedcoin.org/cubatravel/. With that said, we scrambled and miraculously managed to meet the criteria to travel to Cuba "in support of the Cuban people." (This was our actual legal travel category) If I was going to support Cuban people, I was going to be particularly interested in helping Afro-Cubans. The reason being, Afro-Cubans have experienced disenfranchisement and institutional racism, not unlike their African American counterparts. In my efforts to interact with Afro-Cubans as much as possible, I met this Cuban lady, that was just the sweetest soul. She earns a living posing for photos with tourists, but upon further inquiry, she opened up, and we shared a very emotional conversation.

What is the worst travel experience you ever had?

The worst travel experience is inherently connected to my best travel memory because they both happened the first time I traveled. No one forgets their first, neither will I. It was a magical experience filled with wonder and expectation. 'Expectation' is the keyword here. You see, I had watched too many love stories set in Paris and had glamourized the city to unattainable heights. Remember the scene in Casablanca where Bergman's character asks, "what about us?" and Bogart's character replies, "we will always have Paris," as they are saying farewell for good? That was my Paris. Until I got to Paris. We were naive travelers and had planned poorly. As a result, I had a horrid time in there...Travel tip: If you are visiting Paris for the first time, the location you stay at is everything. Invest in centrally located accommodation and budget for taxi fare. Avoid the subway if you can.

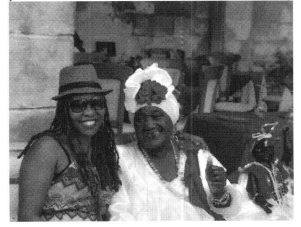

The Ultimate Self-Care Guide for Travelers of Color

Favorite Travel Hack?

Credit Cards! No, I am not suggesting using credit cards to purchase trips you otherwise couldn't afford. I mean using the travel benefits credit cards give you to save big on travel and reap some sweet perks along the way. A good travel credit card should have an awesome miles bonus when you hit a spend amount, zero foreign transaction fees, and numerous other travel rewards, including travel credits and Global Entry fee reimbursement. Yes, some cards will give you money back at the end of the year for travel expenses! We have calculated some credit card annual perks to be in the thousands

What is your travel Ritual for keeping calm and maintaining your inner zen?

I mentioned earlier the idea of making the airport a destination. A lot of people leave the house with just enough time to get to the airport, go through security, and board their flight. Even a slight delay in any part of this process will cause stress levels to spike. Stress is the exact opposite emotion people set out to feel when they plan a vacation. We leave early, allowing more than enough time for unexpected eventualities. If everything goes smoothly, it just means I have some time to spend at the airport. I love exploring the airport shops (They are expensive, but you can find some beautiful souvenirs). Spending time at the airport lounges can be productive and relaxing. Get some work done or relax and have a meal accompanied by a signature fruity cocktail. You will be surprised how stress-free travel can be once you eliminate the rushing and impatience that comes with it.

Best Travel Tip Advice?

I have given travel tips throughout this interview! I have mentioned eliminating the stress of travel by allowing enough time to enjoy the journey and also how you can rip huge rewards by maximizing travel credit card perks. Now that you plan on traveling often be sure to apply for TSA PreCheck or Global Entry. Admission to either of these programs will make life at the airport much less stressful.

Why is addressing mental health in and self-care with as it relates to people of color so important in the travel community?

The black travel community is a pioneering movement that is breaking black stereotypes worldwide. With mantras like "we go too" and "black and abroad," black people everywhere have found representation in a market segment that was notorious for exclusion – the travel industry. Led by smart, creative, and educated individuals, the movement is a trendsetter. This movement now has the attention of young, upwardly mobile black youth, and they are all ears. That is why it is imperative that we, as content creators and leaders of this movement, bring attention to topics that would otherwise be a little taboo among our people. Mental illness is one of the most prevalent yet least talked about diseases among professionals of color. Until we remove the stigma around mental illness and educate our people on why it is as essential to take care of themselves mentally, we shall continue to lose a lot of people to the struggle.

Although we travel often for our mental health, the topic is not emphasized due to shame and stigma. How can we normalize this conversation among the travel communities of color?

A good friend of mine, who is gay, once hypothesized to me that if everybody who was gay came out, the whole world would realize that they all know and love a gay person. I think we can draw the same parallel with mental illness. If everybody struggling with mental health shared their struggles and triumphs, then people would realize how prevalent and "normal" it is and that they are not alone.

Slyvia (Sly) Callendar

WEBSITE

www.twosidedcoin.org

EMAIL

johnandsly@twosidedcoin.org

INSTAGRAM HANDLE

@thetwosidedcoin

FACEBOOK PAGE

facebook.com/twosidedcoin.org

Travel Jokes

THE FIVE LOVE LANGUAGES:

1. **Acts of Service:** *I planned our entire trip.*
2. **Receiving Gifts:** *Here's a trip.*
3. **Quality Time:** *Let's go on a trip together.*
4. **Words of Affirmation:** *You planned a great trip.*
5. **Physical Touch:** *Holding someone's hand on the airplane while on a trip.*

CHAPTER 27

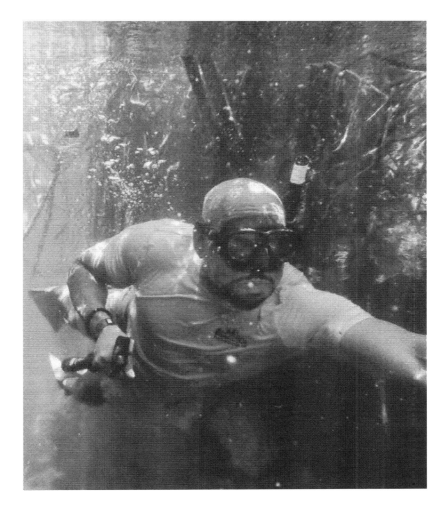

Fanon Wilkins

Epic

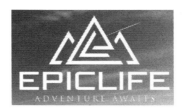

Travel Quote or Travel Mantra you live by
If you are not going to expanding, you are contracting.

How has Traveling helped you maintain your mental health as it relates to self-care?
It's been absolutely essential to recognize the importance of presence and gratitude.

What is your most therapeutic travel destination for stress relief and self-care?
The mountains and the oceans.

Whats is the most important items you have in your carryon and why?
A book. I am a book-aholic. I can go through a book in a week.

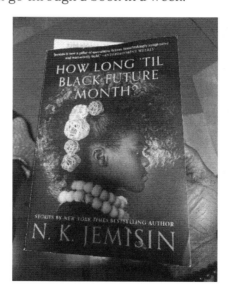

Favorite Calming Beverage or Food to consume while traveling and why?
Water and Nuts. Hydration is key to maintaining good blood circulation on the plane. Nuts are healthy snack food.

Favorite Calming Music or Audio to listen to while traveling?
Oprah's Super Soul Sunday—The Podcast and my Spotify Playlists that include everything from John Coltrane to J. Cole.

Favorite Keepsake that keeps you calm or grounded while traveling?
My Om necklace

Fanon Wilkins

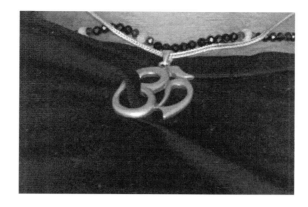

What is your most hilarious travel memory?

Partying in TULUM with 25 of my closest friends on my birthday

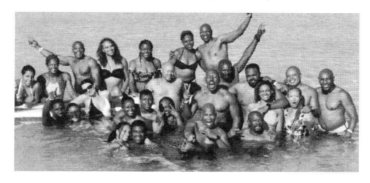

What is your most memorable or touching travel experience?

Two flat tires while bike packing on Victoria Island in B.C., Canada

What is the worst travel experience you ever had?

Van breaking down between Harare, Zimbabwe and Lusaka, Zambia.

Favorite Travel Hack?

Compression bags for my clothes

What is your travel Ritual for keeping calm and maintaining your inner zen?

Presence and Gratitude. Always giving thanks for the opportunity no matter the circumstances.

Best Travel Tip Advice?

Move with an open heart.

Why is addressing mental health in and self-care with as it relates to people of color so important in the travel community?

It's important to dispel the taboo.

Although we travel often for our mental health, the topic is not emphasized due to shame and stigma. How can we normalize this conversation among the travel communities of color?

Through public engagement and the creation of new narratives that are accessible and humanizing.

WEBSITE

epiclifeoutdoors.com

EMAIL

epiclifetraveloutdoorz@gmail.com

INSTAGRAM HANDLE

epiclifeoutdoorz

FACEBOOK PAGE

Epic Life

Travel Jokes

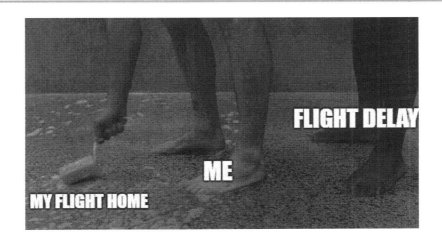

CHAPTER 28

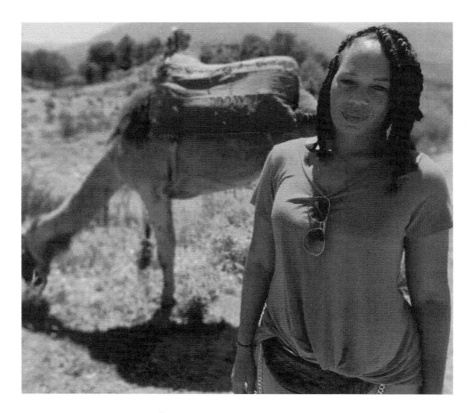

Mahogany Ratcliffe
Duchess of Travel Deals

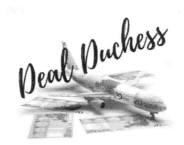

Deal Duchess

Travel Quote or Travel Mantra you live by
Mary J. Blige said it best..."SHARE MY WORLD!"

Travel Influencer/ Brand Summary

Duchess of travel deals and steals. The art of making frugal travel look and feel like a million bucks

How has Traveling helped you maintain your mental health as it relates to self-care?

Travel for me is not only a physical escape but a mental escape. The worries and baggage that I carry are temporarily on hold and the only baggage that is important has wheels and a handle.

What is your most therapeutic travel destination for stress relief and self-care?

Bali for sure! The sunset is incredible. It's a spiritual oasis. I've never been so grateful for nature and existence as I was when I was there.

Whats is the most important items you have in your carryon and why?

Clorox wipes! Planes are absolutely filthy...plus I have to wipe down the hotel toilet...I have visions of them using the same cloth to wipe all toilets.

Favorite Calming Beverage or Food to consume while traveling and why?

I never thought of food as calming. Probably because I eat too much!

Favorite Calming Music or Audio to listen to while traveling?

I listen to a little bit of everything

Favorite Keepsake that keeps you calm or grounded while traveling?

I try to keep it light but a photo of my passport holding traveling baby who is not baby anymore keeps a smile on my face

What is your most hilarious travel memory?

A little boy in Amsterdam following me around calling me Beyonce. Thanks kid, but I'm no Beyonce.

What is your most memorable or touching travel experience?

My mother has wanted to travel to Paris her entire life and I made that happen. It was so amazing to witness her falling in love with what she has always dreamt of.

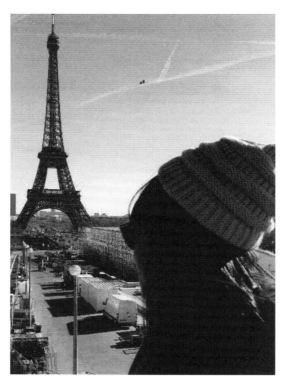

What is the worst travel experience you ever had?

Knock on wood! I haven't had a terrible travel experience and I pray that I never do. I can say, I wasn't wowed by Milan.

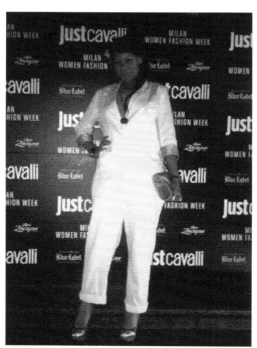

What is your travel Ritual for keeping calm and maintaining your inner zen?

I'm just calm by nature and don't get ruffled easily. I live for adventure and getting lost, so I find what other people get flustered by, fun! Acroyoga with my husband helps!

Favorite Travel Hack

ITA Matrix, Sky Scanner, The Flight Deal

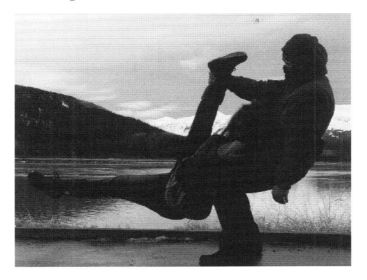

Best Travel Tip Advice?

Money is not the issue, Its knowledge. When you know better, you do better. Sign up to deal duchess so you can receive info on all the flight glitches and amazing flight deals around the world.

Why is addressing mental health in and self-care with as it relates to people of color sc important in the travel community?

Addressing mental health is essential because ignoring what is real becomes a threat and is harmful to our community as a whole. Teaching coping mechanisms is just one way to rid ourselves of many issues that surround us.

Although we travel often for our mental health, the topic is not emphasized due to shame and stigma. How can we normalize this conversation among the travel communities of color?

I think just having a conversation opens doors to healing. Talking with each other is so incredibly therapeutic and that's what's needed.

Travel Jokes

  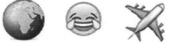

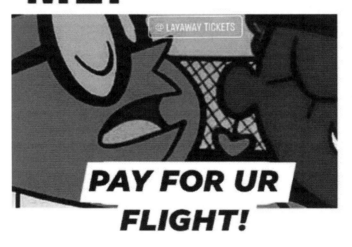

CHAPTER 29

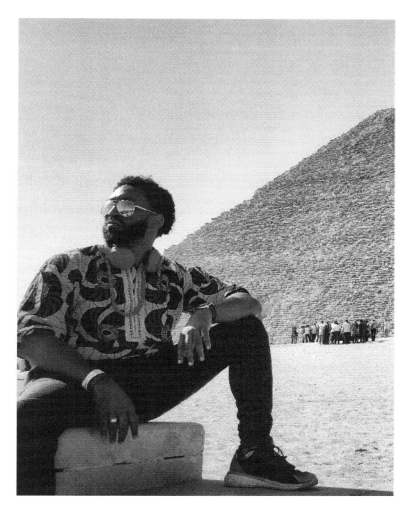

Brett Roberts

Cubicle with Wings

THE PASSPORT BLOG

Travel Quote or Travel Mantra you live by
You only live once, so you might as well live.

How has Traveling helped you maintain your mental health as it relates to self-care?

It provides peace, serenity and escape. I get to learn new things all the time and meet new people. It helps me be a better person who understands and can empathize more when I return from a trip.

What is your most therapeutic travel destination for stress relief and self-care?

Colombia. Great food, culture and people.

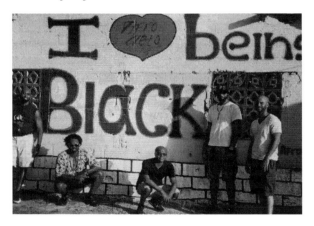

Whats is the most important items you have in your carryon and why?

My chargers, can't do anything without those. My laptop, two portable batteries and my toiletries.

Favorite Calming Beverage or Food to consume while traveling and why?

Green tea or yerba mate.

Favorite Calming Music or Audio to listen to while traveling?

Bachata, Salsa, hip hop, classics and political podcasts.

Favorite Keepsake that keeps you calm or grounded while traveling?

A ring my grandma gave me.

What is your most hilarious travel memory?

Falling out of a canoe into four feet high water on the Dominican Republic but thinking I was going to drown.

Brett Roberts

What is your most memorable or touching travel experience?

> Taking 20 kids to see Black Panther in Colombia.

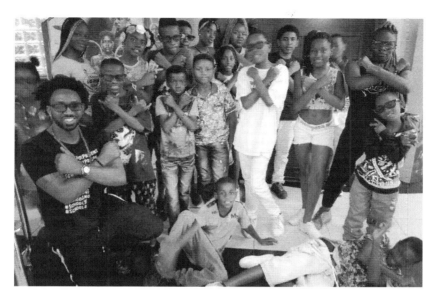

What is the worst travel experience you ever had?

> Having to use the bathroom in the middle of nowhere.

Favorite Travel Hack?

> Using my favorite travel websites to book travel last minute

What is your travel Ritual for keeping calm and maintaining your inner zen?

> I usually make sure that I get a good amount of rest when on the airplane and I know that at the end of the day whether things go right or they go wrong it's all a part of the journey, it's all part of the experience

Best Travel Tip Advice?

> Go far, go often. The only thing that's holding you back is yourself. Don't think about it when it comes to planning a trip, spin the globe point so place and go there.

Why is addressing mental health in and self-care with as it relates to people of color so important in the travel community?

> The images that we see oftentimes on television in the United States can be troubling at best. Watching the nose all the time can put one and a negative place. Venturing out and seeing the world allows for you to see that often psalms what we see is not normal

Although we travel often for our mental health, the topic is not emphasized due to shame and stigma. How can we normalize this conversation among the travel communities of color?

> Healthy non-judgmental conversation

WEBSITE

Www.thepassportblog.com

EMAIL

brettcsroberts@gmail.com

INSTAGRAM HANDLE

@realjetsetbrett

FACEBOOK PAGE

JetSetBrett

Travel Jokes

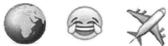

Mf's be scheduling flights, trips and appointments and don't even be having the time off yet... Don't matter because they going anyway 🥷

That's me... I'm mf's

CHAPTER 30

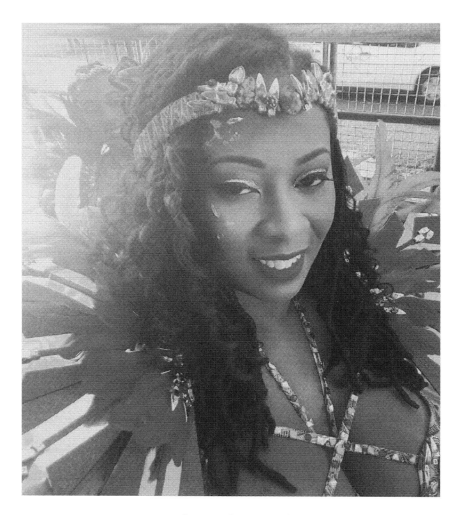

Stephanie Snipes
Carnival Babe

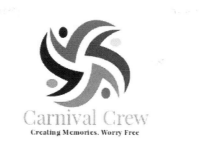

Carnival Crew
Creating Memories, Worry Free

Travel Quote or Travel Mantra you live by
Life is too short to wait until retirement to finally enjoy it.

How has Traveling helped you maintain your mental health as it relates to self-care?

My family has always traveled, even when I was growing up. But I did not start having serious wanderlust until my 30th birthday when my older sister decided to treat me to a birthday trip to Turks and Caicos. That trip help reignite my love of travel, and now as an adult with more monetary means, I was able to explore it in a whole new way. Traveling helped me get through some infertility issues by basically taking my focus away from it. Carnival and traveling have opened up so many doors for me that I did not even plan or could imagine, and my life has been more enriched and stress-free since. This year I was literally sitting in a meeting feeling stressed and bored and said to myself, I can't do this, and booked a last-minute trip to Miami Carnival. I corralled my sisters and cousins to go as well and had the most amazing and stress-free time ever. It helped me come back to work feeling a little more energized.

What is your most therapeutic travel destination for stress relief and self-care?

The tiny but mighty island of Barbados is my home away from home. I try to get there at least twice a year, whether it is an extended stay or long layover that allows me to enjoy the island for 24 hours. Every beach is public there, so you can really take the time to explore. You can find beaches where no one else seems like they exist and just have a moment to yourself and breathe. The people there are very friendly as well, and through my multiple travels there I have made life long friends who are like family and I look forward to seeing every time I go.

Whats is the most important items you have in your carryon and why?

The most important items in my carryon are my makeup bag and my Samsung tablet. I put my makeup in my carryon bag just in case the airline loses my luggage. This way I don't lose my clothes and my face! My tablet is a one-stop-shop for entertainment needs and staying connected in case I need to work on something for my business.

Favorite Calming Beverage or Food to consume while traveling and why?

My favorite calming food to eat while traveling is Corn Soup, a Trinidadian delicacy. Corn soup can easily be found outside of the many fetes (parties) you attend in Trinidad for Carnival. At these fetes you party, eat and drink non-stop for hours. Corn soup nourishes and replenishes you. I've even gotten sick while at Carnival and relied on Corn Soup to make me feel better and get through. If you attend a Carnival event in the US, you can often find a Corn Soup vendor outside, and I've even made it at home (it is that good).

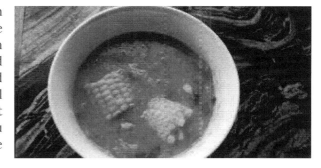

Favorite Calming Music or Audio to listen to while traveling?

Soca is really the only genre of music I listen to these days, whether it is in my car or on a plane. Many people have the misconception that all soca music is "blow your whistle" music, but there are a lot of wonderful groovy/sweet soca songs that are beautiful. This genre also brings me to my happy place, which is at a fete or carnival.

Favorite Keepsake that keeps you calm or grounded while traveling?

My favorite keepsake while traveling is the passport photo of my daughter. If she cannot go on a trip with me, I love having her passport photo with me because it is a reminder that I have already begun to instill my travel and world views into my daughter and I am excited for our adventures ahead, although she cannot come with me always.

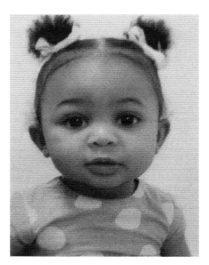

What is your most hilarious travel memory?

Once when I was in middle school, my entire family went to Aruba. We all decided we were going to do an excursion to one of their caves. Now the cave experiences we have had in the past have been underground caves that were cool in temperature with tall cathedral-like ceilings. Not the case in Aruba. First, we came across an entryway that led into a cavern inside the cave. There was a random man in the middle of this cavern and the light on his helmet had gone out. He asked if he could use one of our lamps, and as there were 6 of us we were sure we could give up a lamp. My father walked into that room and when the light showed all around it was full of bats! This was hilarious to me because my father calls himself "The Batman" and yet he was super uncomfortable in the room. But the icing on the cake was when we were trying to get out. This cave was not underground, yet, we had to CLIMB to get out of the cave. We had my grandparents with us so trying to help them get out of the cave led to a lot of funny moments. My grandfather had a really shiny bald head and poor him hit it on one of the rocks trying to climb up and got a nasty cut on top of his head. He was bleeding when we got out, but ultimately okay. We said, whew that was an adventure but we learned our lesson to research our destinations before heading there. We still laugh about our unfortunate adventure to this day.

What is your most memorable or touching travel experience?

My most touching travel experience is when I surprised my mom in Aruba with her best friend who is basically a sister. We had planned a family trip where the best friend was invited but could not afford to go. My mother kept saying to me that it would nice if she could have her there with her. They lived in very far away states at the time and did not get to see each other as often as they would like. So I decided to step in and offer to bring her but kept it a secret. I was able to capture the moment on video when my mom saw her best friend for the first time in Aruba. She was so happy and it brought me so much joy to see them both so happy.

What is the worst travel experience you ever had?

I have been fortunate, even while traveling on an overseas flight with a 1-year-old, to not have had any bad travel experiences. The only thing that really irritated me was the time I missed a connecting flight in Atlanta because my first flight was delayed and my connecting flight was on the other side of the airport. I ran (in flip-flops) dragging a carryon bag all the way across the airport, only to get to the gate, see my plane sitting there, but learn that they had just closed the doors and so could not get me on the flight. A few hours later I was on my way home, but that was the worse and since then, I will not take any flights that connect through ATL.

Favorite Travel Hack?

When booking airfare, if the round trip tickets seem high, I will book in one-way segments. I'll book whichever segment is most important to me and/or cheapest, and then watch the other segment to see if the price drops. Often the price will drop or a layover route that offers the opportunity to see a new destination might come across my way.

What is your travel Ritual for keeping calm and maintaining your inner zen?

On any trip I will find some time for myself to do something that I enjoy, whether it is read a book, take a stroll on the beach or grabbing food from my favorite restaurant if it is a destination I have been before.

Best Travel Tip Advice?

Get a travel reward credit card that you use to pay automatic bills. Pay off the balance every month, but earn those miles/points etc… so that you can use it towards a trip in the future. This may help you travel more often and for less money.

Why is addressing mental health in and self-care with as it relates to people of color so important in the travel community?

People of color, especially those of us from the African Diaspora, deal with microaggressions, institutionalized racism and in your face racism every day. It has been proven that these undercurrents of stress cause PTSD like symptoms in our community and can be passed onto our offspring. In addition to this, if you live in a Western society like the United States, you are living in a hamster wheel of stress. Your life more than likely is consumed by work, bills and family. I do not believe humans were meant to work as long and as much as we are forced to do these days, and it is proven by how many people have anxiety and depression. I think it is important to travel to get the mental break you need from your everyday life. Time to reflect, recharge and reset and come back a better person. Travel also opens you up to new experiences and people, and there may be opportunities and friends that would never come across unless you ventured out into the world.

Although we travel often for our mental health, the topic is not emphasized due to shame and stigma. How can we normalize this conversation among the travel communities of color?

I believe that the younger generations are more open and understanding of Mental Health needs and taking the breaks needed to recoup. As travel influencers and businesses, I think if we continue to speak openly about it in our public forums, then it will become more normalized. I think we should also start conversations in the Corporate world so the stigma of taking a mental health day is removed. If you take time off from work because you are physically ill, most companies are okay with that, especially if it is contagious. Those same attitudes should be carried over for Mental Health.

WEBSITE

www.carnivalcrewvip.com

EMAIL

info@carnivalcrewvip.com

INSTAGRAM HANDLE

carnivalcrewvip

FACEBOOK PAGE

www.facebook.com/carnivalcrewvip

Travel Jokes

Coworker: How many vacation days do you have?

First of all, mind your business.

CHAPTER 31

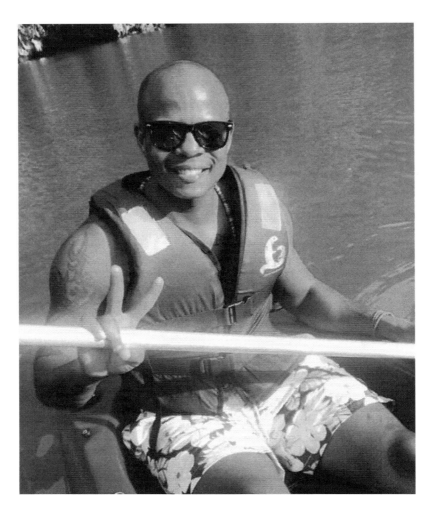

Yahya Bey
TRE Wellness Traveler

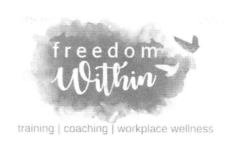

training | coaching | workplace wellness

Travel Quote or Travel Mantra you live by
Meet people where they are.

Travel Influencer/ Brand Summary
Practical wellness solutions for busy professionals

How has Traveling helped you maintain your mental health as it relates to self-care?
Traveling helped create the space needed to get closer to my authentic self and expression.

What is your most therapeutic travel destination for stress relief and self-care?
Nature, anywhere.

Whats is the most important items you have in your carryon and why?
Essential oils. Scents help me to ground.

Favorite Calming Beverage or Food to consume while traveling and why?
Water.

Favorite Calming Music or Audio to listen to while traveling?
Mostly Bach or other classical music.

Favorite Keepsake that keeps you calm or grounded while traveling?
My Nepalese mala necklace

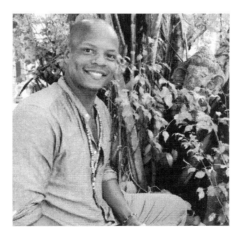

What is your most hilarious travel memory?

>Falling down a volcano in Guatemala.

What is your most memorable or touching travel experience?

>Making the decision not to return to the United States after arriving in Thailand for 3 week holiday and start my own Studio.

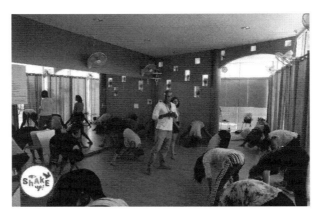

What is the worst travel experience you ever had?

>Have not had any really, most 'worst' experiences usually have something to do with US customs.

Favorite Travel Hack?

>Go. Plan later.

What is your travel Ritual for keeping calm and maintaining your inner zen?

>Nature, Meditation, TRE.

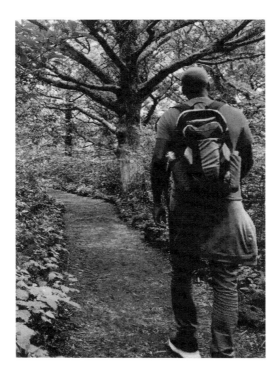

Best Travel Tip Advice?

Explore.

Why is addressing mental health in and self-care with as it relates to people of color so important in the travel community?

Mental health and wellness have reached the point of crisis and need continuous, open and constructive conversations and solutions.

Although we travel often for our mental health, the topic is not emphasized due to shame and stigma. How can we normalize this conversation among the travel communities of color?

Move beyond talking about it. Being proactive about engaging in practices that promote holistic lifestyles, balance and homeostasis. Have honest conversations about lifestyle choices around alcohol to see if they are serving our best interest and promoting positive health choices. More often than not, the answer is simply NO.

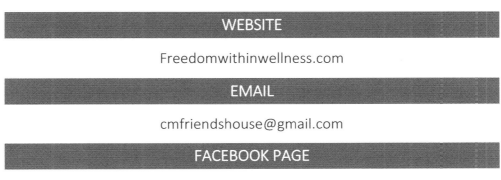

WEBSITE
Freedomwithinwellness.com

EMAIL
cmfriendshouse@gmail.com

FACEBOOK PAGE
YahyaElMajeedBey

Travel Jokes

THE FIVE LOVE LANGUAGES:

1. **Acts of Service:** *I planned our entire trip.*
2. **Receiving Gifts:** *Here's a trip.*
3. **Quality Time:** *Let's go on a trip together.*
4. **Words of Affirmation:** *You planned a great trip.*
5. **Physical Touch:** *Holding someone's hand on the airplane while on a trip.*

CHAPTER 32

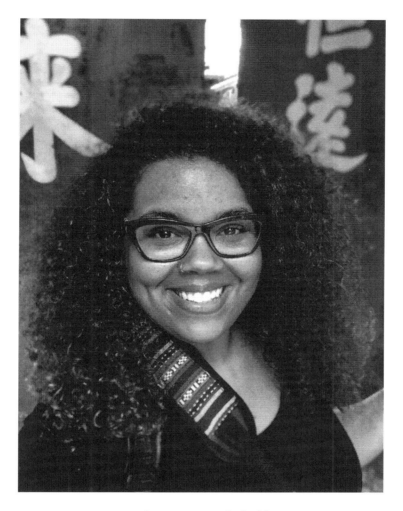

Kristen Riddle

Vibes Travel

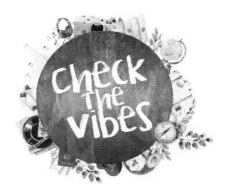

Travel Quote or Travel Mantra you live by
"I think you travel to search and you come back home to find yourself there."
— Chimamanda Ngozi Adichie

How has Traveling helped you maintain your mental health as it relates to self-care?

Before traveling, I could feel myself getting comfortable with the routine. I had a regular 9-5 job, went home, ate, went to sleep just to wake up and do it all again the next day. I wasn't living and that's where travel has helped my mental health. I've never felt freer and at peace with life, and I gained that clarity through my experience with travel.

What is your most therapeutic travel destination for stress relief and self-care?

For now, it'd have to be Krabi, Thailand. Actually, just Thailand in general so far.

Whats is the most important items you have in your carryon and why?

I'll always have my passport, camera, laptop, earplugs & phone. The reason why is because these essentials keep me traveling, as well as in contact with my loved ones back in the states. Plus, I need my laptop and camera to document and write about my experiences on Check the Vibes. The earplugs are for the plane rides. If you know, YOU KNOW. Haha!

Favorite Calming Beverage or Food to consume while traveling and why?

Honestly, I don't have a favorite beverage or food, as I am very open to trying EVERYTHING once. So, street food and the local drinks are my go-to, no matter where I am in the world.

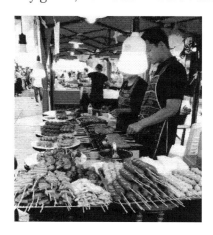

Kristen Riddle

Favorite Calming Music or Audio to listen to while traveling?

Check the Vibes has over 20+ curated playlists on Apple Music as well as Spotify, so, any of those playlists will keep me up and at 'em while on the road.

Favorite Keepsake that keeps you calm or grounded while traveling?

This one is a good one because I always take a few photos with me. A photo of my parents, my sisters and my small group of friends. Whenever I felt homesick, taking a look at them kept my spirits high.

What is your most hilarious travel memory?

Oh my goodness, while in Thailand, I would often get stopped in some parts for people to take pictures. At first, I assumed they thought I was someone I wasn't. Luckily, a local explained to me they aren't used to seeing someone with my hair type in these parts, and the locals found it fascinating. So, they'd stop and ask me for a picture! I felt like a celebrity! Haha!

What is your most memorable or touching travel experience?

My most memorable experience while traveling was the architecture as well as my Sak Yant tattoo ritual I experienced. The buildings in locations all over the world are such a sight to see. Every temple has a meaning. Every building has a different spin on them, and it's a breath of fresh air to see places so different than what I'm used to.

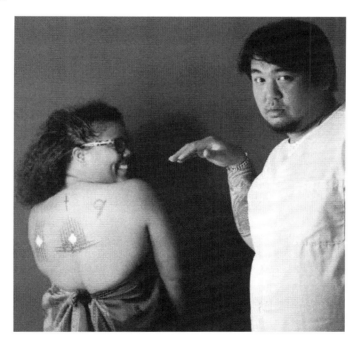

What is the worst travel experience you ever had?

The worst travel experience I've ever had is racism. While in some parts of Thailand, I would have to travel by train. My hair was a lot larger than the norm due to the lack of Black hair-care products in this country, and the humidity didn't help. People would literally move away from me, look at my hair in disgust as well as make faces and SWAT my hair, even if I wasn't close enough to them for my hair to be touching them. Let's just say, hair-wise, I didn't fit the beauty "norm" over there at times.

Favorite Travel Hack?

Talk to the locals! I can't stress this enough. If you're not looking to go to the cliche tourist spots, talk to people around you and see what they have in mind for you to see in their country. You'll discover incredible places this way, and in some cases, you'll make lifelong friends as well.

What is your travel Ritual for keeping calm and maintaining your inner zen?

Oh, this one is easy. My ritual for keeping calm and relaxing while traveling is swimming. I'm a major water baby, so if I encounter the body of water that I can dive into, I will. Being in water allows me to reflect on my blessings.

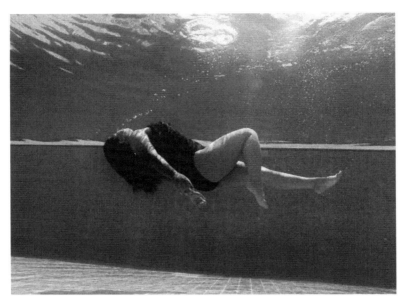

Best Travel Tip Advice?

My best travel advice would be to not be afraid of solo travel. If you wait for someone to travel with you, you may never explore the places you desire. Plan the trip, girl. Get out of your comfort zone, even if you have to do it alone. You will not regret it!

Why is addressing mental health in and self-care with as it relates to people of color so important in the travel community?

It's important to address mental health and self-care for us because no one else will. We're often left out of the conversation when it comes to both mental health and travel, especially by big companies. When traveling solo, we have to speak on the experiences we're dealing with and how we overcome them. I feel travel helps reinvent ourselves as well as put things we're dealing with in the states into perspective. There's a sense of happiness and satisfaction you get while traveling that you're just not able to get in your regular routine. I feel it's important for us to explore that scope.

Although we travel often for our mental health, the topic is not emphasized due to shame and stigma. How can we normalize this conversation among the travel communities of color?

This is a wonderful question because it's so true. I made my first trip due to depression and I was shifted to such a positive mental state almost immediately. Opening the dialogue to this topic and really talking about how our mental health shapes how we live, move and think can only make others more comfortable in talking about it. Even if someone hasn't traveled that much just yet, talking about the state of mental health in our community can be a healing process for so many. It's definitely been a healing process for me.

Kristen Riddle

WEBSITE

https://www.CHECKTHEVIBES.com

EMAIL

kristin@checkthevibes.com

INSTAGRAM HANDLE

https://www.instagram.com/checkthevibes

FACEBOOK PAGE

https://www.facebook.com/checkthevibes

Travel Jokes

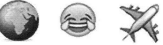

If my bio says my location is Dubai and you happen to see me around, then you are also in Dubai. Let's not complicate things here

CHAPTER 33

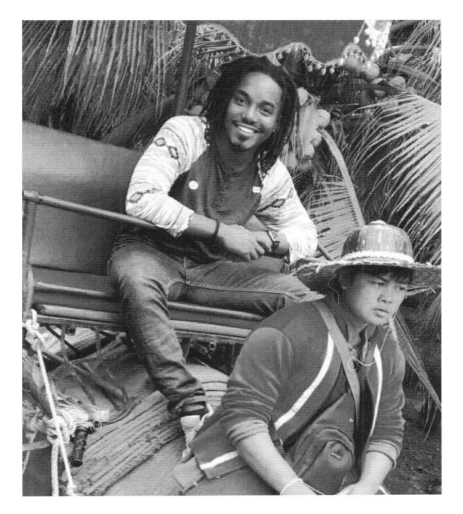

Dr. Keyon Anderson

The Traveling Doctor

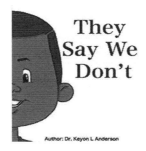

Travel Quote or Travel Mantra you live by
The unknown is scary until it's known.

Travel Influencer/ Brand Summary

Children's Mental Health and Travel Books

How has Traveling helped you maintain your mental health as it relates to self-care?

Travel gives me an opportunity to STOP, take in the world from another lens, and reflect on what's possible.

What is your most therapeutic travel destination for stress relief and self-care?

Jumping in the ocean just outside of Phi Phi Island, Thailand was the most stress relieving/self-care activity I've ever done. As i swim in the water, I felt that I could accomplish all things.

Whats is the most important items you have in your carryon and why?

An essential item in my carryon is my laptop because it allows me to write about my adventures, to stay connected to home and get some work done in real-time.

Favorite Calming Beverage or Food to consume while traveling and why?

Wine!!! Wine is the perfect chill down for almost every destination. The attached picture is from a wine tour I did in Barcelona, Spain.

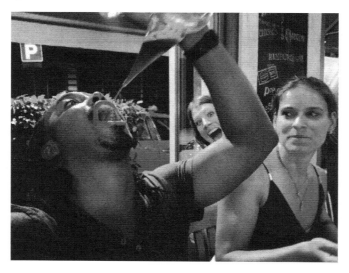

Dr. Keyon Anderson

Favorite Calming Music or Audio to listen to while traveling?

"Walk Thru" by Rich Homie Quan is definitely on the top of my travel playlist, but all in all anything that hypes me up and reminds me to live in the moment.

Favorite Keepsake that keeps you calm or grounded while traveling?

Interesting questions. My bad gave me a stopwatch which I keep in my bag. I've never actually taken a picture of the stopwatch, but it's always close by.

What is your most hilarious travel memory?

I travel with a family friend in China, and everyone thought she was a professional fighter. LOL (Long story and unfortunately there are no pictures)

What is the worst travel experience you ever had?

I don't think I've had any truly awful travel experiences; there are a couple of airlines won't fly and people I won't travel with, but each of these experiences taught me a lot about myself, and I'm thankful.

Favorite Travel Hack?

Pack light and go with the flow. I truly believe that teaches you a lot about yourself and those around you, if you're open and go with the flow.

What is your travel Ritual for keeping calm and maintaining your inner zen?

Download great podcasts (e.g. The Read and Gettin Grown) and bring a couple of great books for long commutes/flights.

Best Travel Tip Advice?

See the silverling in everything that occurs.

Why is addressing mental health in and self-care with as it relates to people of color so important in the travel community?

It is necessary to address mental health and self-care as it relates to people of color in the travel community because we can't just leave our complex identities at home. We take all over who were are with us wherever we go (e.g., our experiences, our oppressions, and our traumas).

Although we travel often for our mental health, the topic is not emphasized due to shame and stigma. How can we normalize this conversation among the travel communities of color?

I think we can normalize talking about mental health/self-care by adding it to the natural flow of conversation. For instance, "How was your trip to.?", "In what ways do you feel refreshed?", "Did you have any moments of clarity or an Ahuh?' We don't need to lead with "How's your mental health now that you took your trip to (blank)."

WEBSITE

keyon.anderson.com

EMAIL

alwaysprogressinginc@gmail.com

INSTAGRAM HANDLE

Dr.Progressing

FACEBOOK PAGE

Keyon Anderson

Dr. Keyon Anderson

Travel Jokes

Alexa, Black Friday travel deal me please

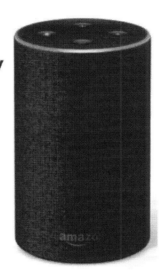

CHAPTER 34

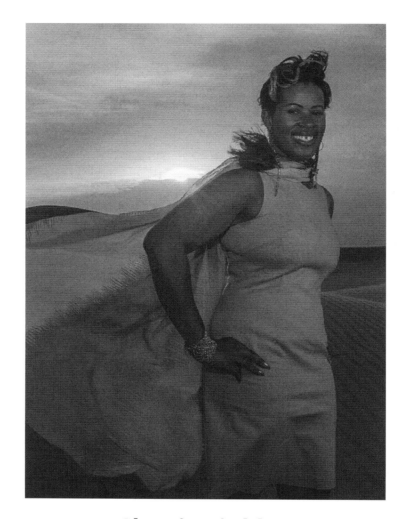

Shani Brinkley

Feeding Your Travel Well

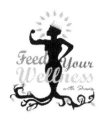

Travel Quote or Travel Mantra you live by
Travel well and travel often.

Travel Influencer/ Brand Summary

Feed your Wellness is a holistic health service provider that customizes wellness initiatives for businesses, private clients, and school systems. We produce inspired events, workshops and develop children's health and well-being programs. We executive produce the Women's F.I.T. Show Wellness Experience in Abu Dhabi. The event uplifts women promotes lifestyle changes through positive mental health and wellness. Produced currently since 2017, women have created new self-care routines, involved family in healthy activities resulting in better mental healthcare.

How has Traveling helped you maintain your mental health as it relates to self-care?

Traveling exposes me to cultures and experiences outside of my normal every day. It reminds me to express gratitude for being able to travel. Being in a state of thankfulness opens up unlimited possibilities and offers a deeper perspective. As the daughter of former Peace Corps' volunteer teachers, I learned at a young age the importance of extending my learning and spiritual development outside of my normal environment. When I traveled now my focus is on increasing my wellness practices. I look for ways to try out new self-care rituals. In some ways, it is why I choose to go to a certain country. For example, one of the reasons I went to Budapest was because of the medicinal thermal pools. In Sri Lanka, we spent time in reverence for elephants. With each trip, my mental health has been supported and reinforced with a deeper practice of self-care.

What is your most therapeutic travel destination for stress relief and self-care?

Phuket, Thailand. My daughter and I went to a wellness retreat. We detoxed for 5 days and exercised for 5 days. It was the perfect setting for self-care. The beach, the mountains, healthy food, mediation and Muay-Thai boxing all lent itself to self-care. We had to turn inward and focus on listening to what our bodies needed, what was missing and how to nurture it. I highly recommend wellness retreats.

Whats is the most important items you have in your carryon and why?

My rosewater spray because I love the smell of roses. When I spray it I immediately feel loved and whole

Favorite Calming Beverage or Food to consume while traveling and why?

Hot cinnamon water. I carry cinnamon sticks and my thermos. Just adding hot water to the sticks and allowing it to percolate, it creates the sweetest, warmest beverage, I feel warm and cozy after drinking it.

Favorite Calming Music or Audio to listen to while traveling?

Sound therapy bowls. My Spotify playlist by Maryam Hasnaa, it reprograms my mind to expect great things to happen.

Favorite Keepsake that keeps you calm or grounded while traveling?

> My journal called Thoughts Along the Way. My former client created it as a result of our work together. The journal is amazing. I record how I'm feeling, my thoughts about my trip and etc. Afterward, I can reflect on my experiences.

What is your most hilarious travel memory?

> Being "proposed" to in Greece. This funny guy kept proposing to me, he was hilarious in his antics.

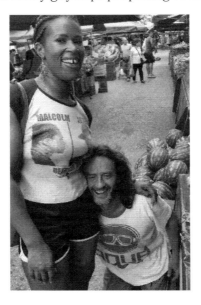

What is your most memorable or touching travel experience?

> Visiting an orphanage in Zanzibar. My daughter instantly connected with the babies. We both felt a deep sense of gratitude.

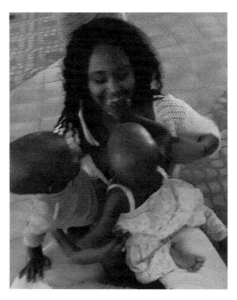

What is the worst travel experience you ever had?

> Throwing up repeatedly on the way up the mountain in Bali. My driver didn't understand English, so I couldn't tell him to pull over. I felt so bad. It was the worst case of car sickness ever.

Shani Brinkley

Favorite Travel Hack?

Take the stairs whenever you can. Try a bike tour or walking tour to easily get exercise in.

What is your travel Ritual for keeping calm and maintaining your inner zen?

Breathing. 4 long breaths are transformative. My body chemistry changes and I immediately calm down.

Best Travel Tip Advice?

Create your own travel experience. Don't be afraid to travel solo. Be safe and do your research.

Why is addressing mental health in and self-care with as it relates to people of color so important in the travel community?

Self-care for us has been almost an act of revolution. We are taught to care for others before caring for ourselves. Therefore, putting ourselves first is an act of rebellion. As people of color, it is necessary for us to put ourselves first and care for our needs. Always giving to others depletes our energy resulting in enormous stress and repressed emotions. It's killing us slowly. Mental health and self-care have to be taught to our communities for our survival.

Although we travel often for our mental health, the topic is not emphasized due to shame and stigma. How can we normalize this conversation among the travel communities of color?

We normalize mental health by having more conversations and being vulnerable. Sharing our collective struggles and triumphs with mental health helps all of us. It normalizes mental awareness.

WEBSITE

www.feedyourwell.info

EMAIL

Shanibrinkley@gmail.com

INSTAGRAM HANDLE

ShaniHealthspark

FACEBOOK PAGE

Feed Your Well

Travel Jokes

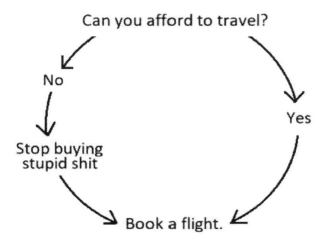

CHAPTER 35

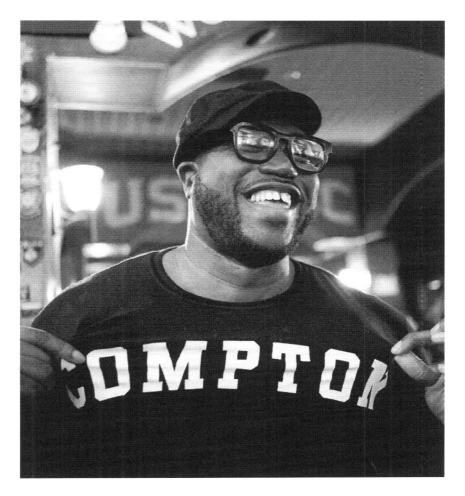

Michael Agyin

Traveling While Deaf

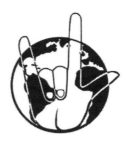

Travel Quote or Travel Mantra you live by

Just because you can't hear the world doesn't mean
You can't explore it.

Travel Influencer/ Brand Summary

Positive Images and Inclusion of Traveling While Deaf

How has Traveling helped you maintain your mental health as it relates to self-care?

Traveling the world through running has helped me to maintain my mental health by allowing me to see the world in ways that I explore it with such a visual effect appreciating the sites the colors the culture the food anything and everything that reminds me there so much to see and do that how can I ever get bored when I travel. The opportunity to reset mentally and also proving that a person with a disability can travel on his/her own and be safe makes me feel whole that anything I put my mind to everything is possible.

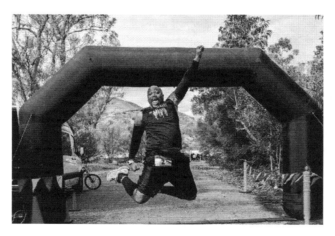

What is your most therapeutic travel destination for stress relief and self-care?

As a more domestic traveler and Travel Runner, the most therapeutic travel destination for stress relief and self-care has been Hawaii for me. The blue oceans the laid back culture the native peoples and the cross-cultural traditions and foods and most importantly I can be still I can sit by the ocean all alone and feel every vibration as I'm one with the island and for that moment I'm at peace.

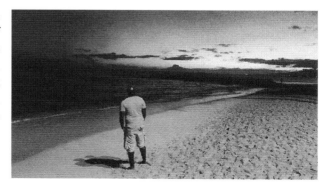

Michael Agyin

Whats is the most important items you have in your carryon and why?

This might sound trivial but my cellphone charger I do a lot over my phone and it's a lifeline to dealing with the hearing world. I have access to things I need such as texting, Google, an app to use for communication with others, uber/lyft apps VP phone to call using an online ASL interpreter so I need to stay connected so my travel experiences stay pleasant and make me less dependent on others for help

Favorite Calming Beverage or Food to consume while traveling and why?

My favorite calming beverage is getting ginger ale anything with ginger has smoothing properties for me and I like to get a drink in mid-air to kinda give me a lil kick to enjoy the flight.

Favorite Calming Music or Audio to listen to while traveling?

Since I'm deaf I listen to music differently since I feel the music not hear the music, the irony is loud hip hop music actually gets me calm but also hyped up! Like here we go to a new adventure we go!! Right now Kenrick Lamar All the Stars is my go-to song when I wanna get ready to travel or then again get hyped!

Favorite Keepsake that keeps you calm or grounded while traveling?

My favorite keepsake is a rubberband I wear that keeps me clam and that I can do this ie. Travel on my own etc the rubberband has the words inscribed "I'm unbreakable" it's really my never give up the mantra and keeps me grounded when things hit the fan especially when I travel or in a new setting etc.

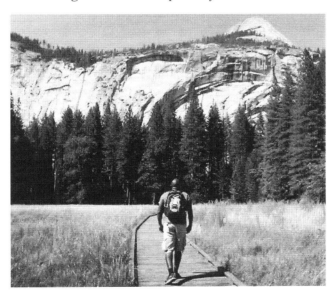

What is your most hilarious travel memory?

One of the most hilarious travel memories was I actually got on the wrong flight and ended up in another state that wasn't my destination! Apparently, I didn't know they made a gate change and the airline staff didn't double-check my ticket so by the time we all realize it was a mistake we were already in the air! It wasn't funny then but It's funny now.. and nowadays on double even triple making sure I'm on the right flight before I even take a seat anywhere!!

What is your most memorable or touching travel experience?

This was very recently but one of the most memorable travel experiences was able to fly into Springfield Massachusetts with my mom. The reason this was memorable as it was my 1st trip to the city I was born in, 34 years. I had left Springfield when I was like 5 years old so it was a trip to see places I've only remembered from pictures when I was a kid to seeing the hospital I was born at to the where my mom used to work or the places we used to go to and I felt a sense of knowing a part of me has been made whole by going home. It was by far one of the best trips I've been able to experience!

What is the worst travel experience you ever had?

The worst travel experience I ever had was needing to take 4 different flights in one day just to get to a really small airport in Redding California! Went from LAX to Arizona, to San Francisco to Redding and it was so confusing because I'm not sure what's going on since info was sent through a speakerphone and nobody told me there was going to be all these layovers and flight changes so I really had to find a way to communicate with airline staff and have people write down information because it became an all-day affair and I ended up getting to my destination super late at night then having to figure out how to get from the airport to my destination that wasn't in the actual area and this was before uber/ lyft was available!

Favorite Travel Hack?

My favorite travel hack is knowing all the low-cost airlines directly so when I'm looking for a flight I can get the information straight from the source rather than an app or 3 parties and it helps some of these airlines know me so when I'm at the airport airline staff know what to do..and more frequently I've been introduced to staff that now know sign language! I also keep a frequent miles account so I can get points to get free/cheap flights from time to time.

What is your travel Ritual for keeping calm and maintaining your inner zen?

My travel ritual for keeping calm and maintaining my inner zen is making sure I arrive to the airport early enough that I have time to deal with anything that pops up and as a deaf person I know it's better to deal with an issue at the airport rather than the over the phone which would be a total failure, basically I keep an open mind that anything can happen but learn to take everything in stride. Keep calm and carrying on

Best Travel Tip Advice?

As a person with a disability, my best travel tip is to know and understand your rights as a traveler! Can't stress this enough. You have the right to access information for all your travel needs. If you have physical disabilities etc you have the right to make sure they handle your wheelchair/ equipment with care and above all you deserve respect and dignity just like any other passenger who travels! So know your travel rights

Why is addressing mental health in and self-care with as it relates to people of color so important in the travel community?

This is so important because many of us come from backgrounds where traveling wasn't important and never taking a break from their reality. Travel experiences really to provide a place to decompress and grow by expanding and exploring the world outside your comfort zone and challenges you to think creatively and passionately about what and how yo do when you travel to places that can also enlightened you, and for people of color this the best kind of growth you can ask for.

Although we travel often for our mental health, the topic is not emphasized due to shame and stigma. How can we normalize this conversation among the travel communities of color?

I believe we can normalize this by being open-minded and practicing inclusion that was all dealing with something and the more we act like a community that shares and using travel as way to become whole as a person will lead to a stronger and interwoven community that encourages everyone to be open and foster a safe space in which our travels become like healing energy that works from within.

Michael Agyin

EMAIL

mkagyin@yahoo.com

INSTAGRAM HANDLE

mikeyisjusssayin

FACEBOOK PAGE

Michael Agyin

Travel Jokes

  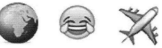

Does anyone else pack underwear like they're going to s**t themselves every single day of a trip?

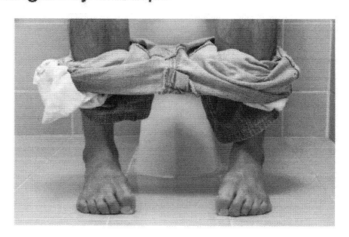

CHAPTER 36

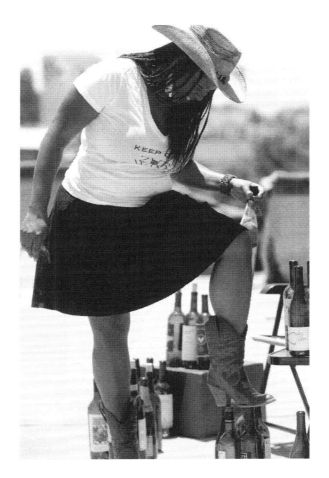

Tuanni Price

Wine Tours

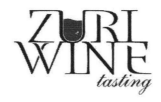

Travel Quote or Travel Mantra you live by
Live Like a Local and always bring wine

How has Traveling helped you maintain your mental health as it relates to self-care?
Yes it resets my values and helps me to appreciate life

What is your most therapeutic travel destination for stress relief and self-care?
Cape Town South Africa

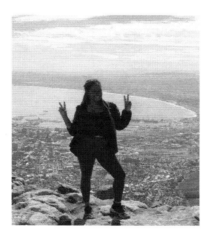

Whats is the most important items you have in your carryon and why?
Change of underwear, face wipes, moisturizer and a journal.

Favorite Calming Beverage or Food to consume while traveling and why?
Wine Wine Wine and More Wine

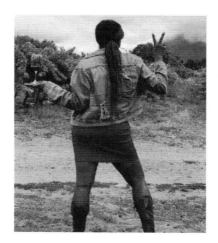

Tuanni Price

Favorite Calming Music or Audio to listen to while traveling?

    Neo-soul & my podcast

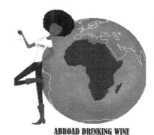

Favorite Keepsake that keeps you calm or grounded while traveling?

    A necklace with an egg that opens with a bird in it. My mother gave it to me when I first moved to Cape Town for a long term stay

What is your most hilarious travel memory?

    Being chased by police while in a taxi bus

What is your most memorable or touching travel experience?

    Teaching at PYDA and having the students show such appreciate

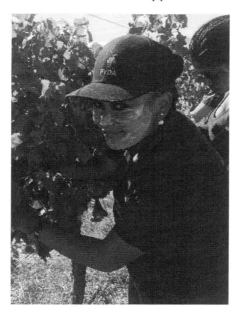

What is the worst travel experience you ever had?

    Being stuck in Paris without a hotel room when a friend of a friend decided last minute that I could not stay at their place

Favorite Travel Hack?

    Hooper

What is your travel Ritual for keeping calm and maintaining your inner zen?

Prayer

Best Travel Tip Advice?

Treat locals with respect. Be kind and aware

Why is addressing mental health in and self-care with as it relates to people of color so important in the travel community?

Treating mental health is important because it is often time overlooked.

Although we travel often for our mental health, the topic is not emphasized due to shame and stigma. How can we normalize this conversation among the travel communities of color?

More conversations about stress and triggers would help

WEBSITE

zuriwine.com

EMAIL

zuriwine@gmail.com

INSTAGRAM HANDLE

tuanniprice

FACEBOOK PAGE

Tuanni Price

Travel Jokes

My next relationship: sex and trips. We just gonna be cumming and going.

CHAPTER 37

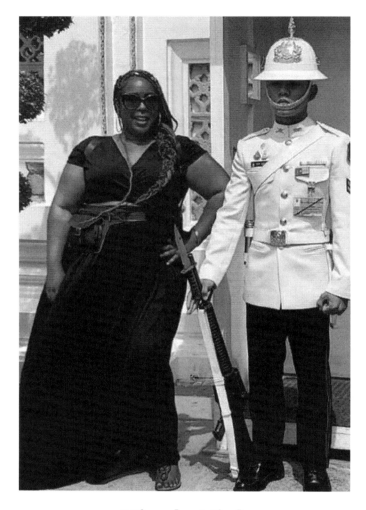

Nicole Vick

Travel Sytles

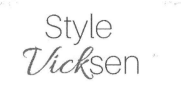

Travel Quote or Travel Mantra you live by
"You must do the thing you think you cannot do."
- Eleanor Roosevelt

Travel Influencer/ Brand Summary

Nicole Vick, also known as Style Vicksen, is a fashion/beauty blogger with a Southern California perspective. She has always been excited about fashion (especially vintage clothes) and nails and can trace her love for fashion and beauty back to her great grandmother and grandmother. Ms. Vick also has a love for supporting local businesses owned by black women. She believes that there is immense talent and expertise in South Central Los Angeles that is incredibly valuable and should be shared with the masses.

How has Traveling helped you maintain your mental health as it relates to self-care?

Traveling is such an important part of mental health maintenance and self-care. The literal and figurative aspect of leaving home, work, stress, and all other troubles behind to find peace and quiet or adventure is wonderful. As a public health professional, I know very well how detrimental chronic stress can be on the body and how important it is to find ways to mitigate that stress to avoid health events like heart attack and stress. For many black people, travel can be a privilege that is both unattainable and very foreign, so the very act of "getting away" can be a true act of defiance, rebellion, courage, and commitment that is absolutely necessary and life-saving.

What is your most therapeutic travel destination for stress relief and self-care?

I am very new to international travel, so I don't have much experience in that realm, but in my late 20s and early 30s I used to make sure I took small trips to Vegas and Palm Springs from time to time. However, the most important trips that I took for stress relief and self-care were the mini-vacations I took to Calabasas. I would use sites like hotwire.com to find cheap hotels and getaway for the weekend by myself. I would pretend I was a tourist and go sightseeing, visit the spa, order room service, and really take time to be alone in my own thoughts. Those were the most inexpensive trips, but the most effective trips.

Whats is the most important items you have in your carryon and why?

I have a few items in my carryon that I think are very important. The first is my medication. I have strong anxiety on long flights and I need medication to help even out my mood and to help me relax. The second most important thing are my noise-canceling headphones. The third most important is my tablet. I download Netflix movies and Spotify tunes so that I have things to occupy my time. All three items saved my life while traveling internationally for the first time. I had so much fear and anxiety about leaving the country leading up to the trip. As the trip grew closer, the fear grew ever more present. I had gotten all the comforting words I was going to get from others. I had to give myself the rest. I realized that the only way to get over it, was to go through it. I had to do it for myself, even if I honestly thought I wouldn't make it back home. Thankfully all the tips worked and I enjoyed my trip!

Favorite Calming Beverage or Food to consume while traveling and why?

Hot tea is probably the most calming beverage for me. Familiar foods are also great, but not always attainable for me since I'm vegan. It can be really hard to find vegan food in many airports or other travel areas. I usually go for cashews, popcorn, or hummus while traveling. Very easy to find and I don't have to worry if they're vegan or not.

Favorite Calming Music or Audio to listen to while traveling?

I enjoyed the Airplane playlist on Spotify. The music was nice and calming and it helped me relax. Also listening to my "sleep" playlists also helped me relax as well. I listened to Masego as well. I like his music a lot and it helped to have music that reminded me of home.

Favorite Keepsake that keeps you calm or grounded while traveling?

I can't say that I have a favorite keepsake while traveling. I'd be so afraid that I'd lose it.

What is your most hilarious travel memory?

I once went with a friend to Vegas years ago and we got invited to a frat party. I was told that it would be crazy and wild. It was not as wild or freaky deeky as I imagined. The party was pretty tame. I've since experienced parties that were more in line with what I was expecting to see that day.

What is your most memorable or touching travel experience?

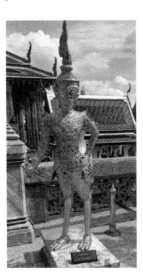

My most memorable experience was visiting the beautiful temples of Bangkok. They were all so very ornate and majestic! I enjoyed taking in all the beautiful sights and learning about the culture while I was there. I will never forget my time there. The second most memorable experience was getting clothes made while there. I felt like a rich girl.

What is the worst travel experience you ever had?

I drove with a friend to Palm Springs and for some reason decided to make the drive without my glasses. Bad decision. By the time we arrived, I had the worst headache ever and it lasted the entire trip. I spent the whole time in Palm Springs in the bed. My friend was not happy at all. I felt bad but I couldn't do anything with my headache.

Favorite Travel Hack?

I haven't found any yet!

What is your travel Ritual for keeping calm and maintaining your inner zen?

Klonopin is definitely part of my keep calm ritual, especially when I'm flying long distances. Other than that, a lot of self-talk works for me. Music also helps to keep me calm. I'll sing to myself to keep me centered.

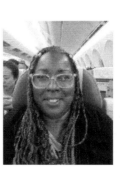

Best Travel Tip Advice?

Just do it! Travel with friends if possible.

Why is addressing mental health in and self-care with as it relates to people of color so important in the travel community?

It's very important for the travel community to address mental health and self-care for black people. The reality is that black people are often in lower socioeconomic status, so travel is simply not a reality for them. We have to think about how to introduce these concepts to people that might not think that travel is a possibility

Nicole Vick

Although we travel often for our mental health, the topic is not emphasized due to shame and stigma. How can we normalize this conversation among the travel communities of color?

The only way to normalize these types of conversations is to continue to have them. We have to talk about mental health until it becomes.

WEBSITE

www.stylevicksen.com

EMAIL

vicksen@stylevicksen.com

INSTAGRAM HANDLE

@stylevicksen

FACEBOOK PAGE

https://www.facebook.com/stylevicksen/

Travel Jokes

Idk who need to hear this but that shirt you looking for is in that suitcase you still haven't unpacked from yo last trip...

CHAPTER 38

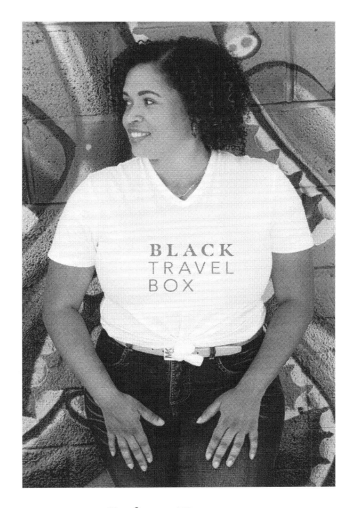

Orion Brown

Black Travel in a Box

BLACK TRAVEL BOX

Travel Quote or Travel Mantra you live by
"Travel changes you. As you move through this life and this world you change things slightly, you leave marks behind, however small. And in return, life – and travel – leaves marks on you. Most of the time, those marks – on your body or on your heart – are beautiful."
Anthony Bourdain

How has Traveling helped you maintain your mental health as it relates to self-care?

Oh my, after 15 years in corporate America I've learned that taking vacation time and seeing a broader lens of the world regularly really helped me to stay grounded, reconnect with God and other people, and kept me from being jaded.

What is your most therapeutic travel destination for stress relief and self-care?

Croatia – mountains, beaches, kind people, and great (healthy too!) seafood.

Whats is the most important items you have in your carryon and why?

I always keep a co-wash or conditioner bar with me, a basic hair and scalp moisturizer, and a detangling comb. That way I'm covered if I need a quick hair refresh, even with protective styles. Of course, I love my brand BlackTravelBox for cleansing and conditioning. And my favorite travel comb is by Ouidad (not pictured).

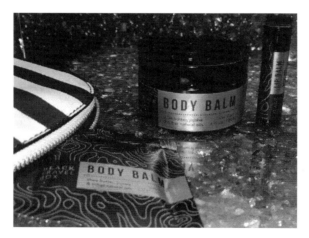

Favorite Calming Beverage or Food to consume while traveling and why?

I really love to eat, so that's a hard one to nail down. But one thing I do like to do in every country I go to is trying their local beer. It makes me feel like a local and its a great conversation starter to learn more about the local culture and history. You can learn a lot through the lore of where and how a national beverage came about. (photo from Bali)

Orion Brown

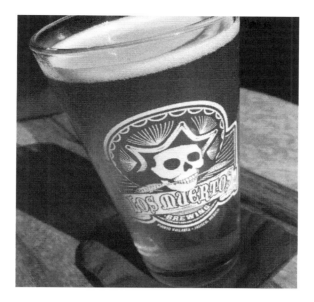

Favorite Calming Music or Audio to listen to while traveling?

Tidal has a great Hip-hop Tranquilo playlist that I love to keep on loop for longer flights. It's got a lot of chill beats but still keeps me feeling soulful. I'm also a fan of Jidenna's Boomerang album – its short, but mixes some really classic melodies with modern beats in a way that makes me feel really cool (and calm!) walking through the busy airport 😊

Favorite Keepsake that keeps you calm or grounded while traveling?

I don't like to take anything I'm not willing to lose (you never know!), but I have kept these photo booth pics of me with family and friends in my wallet for years, at this point they pretty much travel with me everywhere.

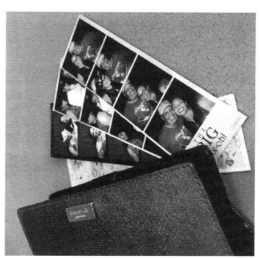

What is your most hilarious travel memory?

I was in Kenya with Habitat for Humanity building a home in Homa Bay – and the local women made us lunch daily. It was amazing BTW! So everyone in our group was basically playing not-it on the chicken head that was included in the stew. I decided to claim it and have a little fun 😊

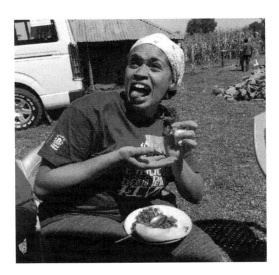

What is your most memorable or touching travel experience?

In 2010, I went to the top of Table Mountain in South Africa. It was absolutely breathtaking and the first time I had ever been that high up and didn't feel afraid. I can't explain why, but what would normally be a white-knuckled, anxiety-ridden excursion for me became the most grounding and comforting moment I've ever experienced on a trip. It was a life-changing moment of gratitude.

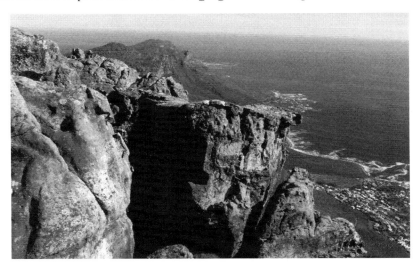

What is the worst travel experience you ever had?

Ah! I've purged the bad and only left the good. But what I will say is this... be willing to get lost, try something that seems gross, and talk to strangers. Everything that's been a 'bad' experience for me had nothing to do with taking risks.

Favorite Travel Hack?

Fill packing cubes based on the itinerary. So for instance, I'll have a cube for clothes to change into when I arrive, dinner that night, and that night's PJs. That way I don't have to fully unpack the luggage to find things when I need them. Also, if I end up checking luggage I'll use that day 1 packing cube in my carry on just in case the luggage gets lost or delayed.

What is your travel Ritual for keeping calm and maintaining your inner zen?

Find a sunrise or sunset and quietly watch it. Daily if possible. And listening to music during any commuting – it gives a soundtrack to the experience (which makes for nice memories) and allows me to really focus on taking in the surroundings rather than being distracted with chatter and noise.

Best Travel Tip Advice?

If you really want to go to as many places as you can, try to create flexibility in your schedule so you can take advantage of deals when they happen. Some of my best trip experiences and deals were with less than two weeks' notice. Sick days work great for this;-P Favorite travel deal sites – Scotts Cheap Flights and Travelzoo

Why is addressing mental health in and self-care with as it relates to people of color so important in the travel community?

I think a big reason we have a Black travel community is the need for self-care. We're finding our own sense of escapism while also using travel to re-discover ourselves. Travel expands our perspective, renews our sense of wonder, and often times acts as a relief to the daily pressures of being a person of color in the US. While not every trip is perfect, it's a much-needed release. So having conversations about the benefits of travel as self-care and also how we can better leverage the experiences in our own mental and emotional health journeys is vital to helping the community get the most out of their travel experiences.

Although we travel often for our mental health, the topic is not emphasized due to shame and stigma. How can we normalize this conversation among the travel communities of color?

I think we do talk about it, it's just more tongue in cheek. We do express being relieved or getting away from work, kids, and people's 'b.s.'. I think what is missing is an acknowledgment that the break is not just because we're 'fed up' but that our ability to be at our best is on the line – our emotional health is on the line. So prioritizing the time away isn't a frivolous thing – its an imperative to enable us to better cope. Normalizing the conversation is a matter of saying we all feel and experience these stresses and we all need a break.

WEBSITE

www.theblacktravelbox.com

EMAIL

orion@theblacktravelbox.com

INSTAGRAM HANDLE

theblacktravelbox

FACEBOOK PAGE

Theblacktravelbox

Travel Jokes

When the whole squad cancels but you're strong, independent young person who don't need no friends.

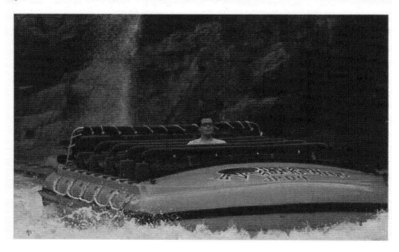

CHAPTER 39

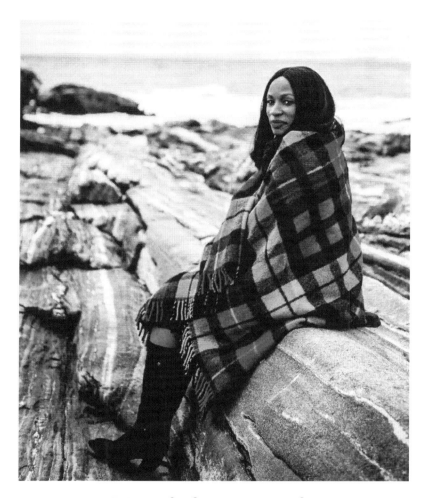

Martinique Lewis

Fighting for Diversity in Travel

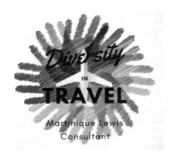

Travel Quote or Travel Mantra you live by
I haven't been everywhere yet, but it's on my list.

Travel Influencer/ Brand Summary

Martinique Lewis is diversity in travel consultant, content creator and Influencer Manager. Trusted amongst her peers as a "connector" she is always connecting the dots to ensure the travel industry is mindful of diversity and not just as a 'Buzz word".Working with numerous tourism boards and travel brands she is constantly strategizing ways to ensure travel marketing campaigns are inclusive and all travelers feel represented. As an international speaker, her goal has always been the same, to change the face of tourism forever.

How has Traveling helped you maintain your mental health as it relates to self-care?

Sometimes we need a mental break from all the things going on in our extremely busy lives. Sometimes I am at most peace in a country nobody even knows about, locked in all day. My sanity is most important!

What is your most therapeutic travel destination for stress relief and self-care?

For me its Trinidad, and during carnival!!! Lol. I know a lot of people would be surprised, but I call Carnival my new year because of its so many beautiful people, the best music, beautiful colors and good vibes only! But even if you went to Trinidad or Tobago outside of Carnival it's so stress-free. Especially Tobago! It's so quiet and calm and easy living, away from the noise etc.

Whats is the most important items you have in your carryon and why?

Acts of Faith by Iyanla Vanzant, I need my daily dose of gratitude and encouragement. My international charger because I have no idea where I'll end up. My Camera, to be able to capture the true essence, not for social media, but for myself. When you are a self-proclaimed photographer you notice the beauty even in the strangest places.

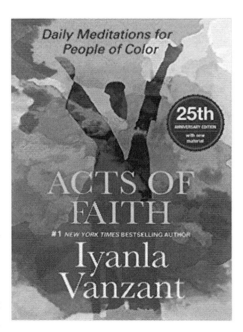

Favorite Calming Music or Audio to listen to while traveling?

Any Soca Music, and then the rest depends on where I am lol. Stormzy Blinded by your grace is my go-to whenever I touch down in London Town. Happy Face by Destiny's child is a go-to. Burna Boy Ye is my jam. But any Soca Chune for sure.

Favorite Keepsake that keeps you calm or grounded while traveling?

A rock from my mom that says I believe in you. She got me the rock to be my gratitude rock. If you've ever watched the secret, there's a portion in there that talks about a gratitude rock. It's a rock that reminds you of all the reasons you have to be grateful, and every time you pick it up you say something you are grateful for.

What is your most hilarious travel memory?

I don't think I have one, lol. My memories are not really funny, I need to work on that!

What is your most memorable or touching travel experience?

My birthday this year. I traveled to Cartagena for my birthday and I was doing a giveback with the Alex Rocha youth center. We brought the kid's school supplies and wanted to play with them so we did. And they were so thoughtful and got me a birthday cake. It surprised me. Even though we don't speak the same language they thought of me enough to go out of their way to celebrate me. It brought me to tears and was one of the best feelings I've ever felt.

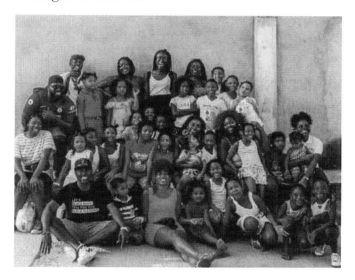

What is the worst travel experience you ever had?

I'm lucky to say I don't have one, and never plan on being able to answer this question.

Favorite Travel Hack?

Mobile passport! Lord, I am so thankful for it. Upon returning to the U.S. if you don't have global entry, a mobile passport is quicker and no one is ever in that line. You fill out everything on your app, and scan your phone and go, I'm literally in baggage claim 7 minutes after landing back in the U.S.

What is your travel Ritual for keeping calm and maintaining your inner zen?

Waking up, giving thanks, and reading Acts of Faith.

Best Travel Tip Advice?

use Facebook groups to help you find people that look like you. Everyone wants to see themselves in the destinations they visit.

Why is addressing mental health in and self-care with as it relates to people of color so important in the travel community?

Because we don't discuss it EVER. Like it's forbidden or something. Sometimes you leaving is the only way to find yourself! Your likes, dislikes, perspective and even love. When you are complacent in only your habitat that's a problem, there's more than the world needs to offer you. Places where you can think,

The Ultimate Self-Care Guide for Travelers of Color

places that bring you joy. Introduce you to perfect strangers and connects you to communities who are intrigued by you. Free your mind.

Although we travel often for our mental health, the topic is not emphasized due to shame and stigma. How can we normalize this conversation among the travel communities of color?

Continue to speak about it through events like audacity fest and books like this. We leaders must lead and show the real sides that may not be popular on social media, but will save a life! It's up to us.

WEBSITE

www.martysandiego.com

EMAIL

marty@abctravelnetwork.com

INSTAGRAM HANDLE

@marty_sandiego

Travel Jokes

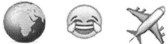

Popeye's Chicken Sandwich is for people that act fancy flying first class on Spirit.

CHAPTER 40

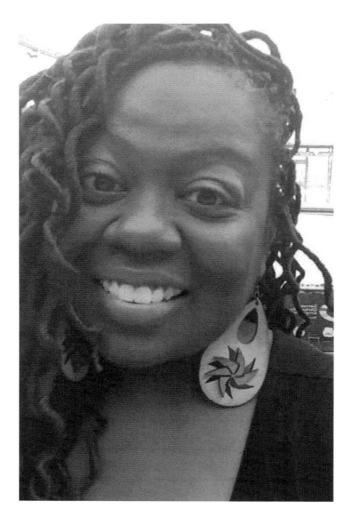

Tammy Freeman
Brazil Soul Story

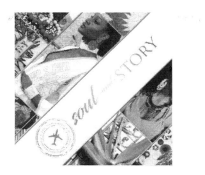

Travel Quote or Travel Mantra you live by

"Travel isn't always pretty. It isn't always comfortable. Sometimes it hurts, it even breaks your heart. But that's okay. The journey changes you; it should change you. It leaves marks on your memory, on your consciousness, on your heart, and on your body. You take something with you. Hopefully, you leave something good behind." — Anthony Bourdain

Travel Influencer / Brand Summary

Telling stories of social entrepreneurs around the world. I work in the world of social impact and I pursue economic justice. An advocate for global citizenship, a world where we do good individually, but better collectively.

How has Traveling helped you maintain your mental health as it relates to self-care?

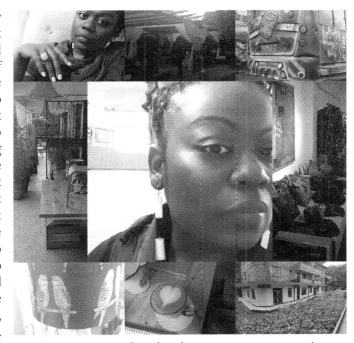

Travel has allowed me to step back from my daily life, evaluate it and learn about what I truly want for my life and what I value. People love to travel because it is a reprieve from the daily hustle of life. From bills, from responsibilities, from traffic and dead-end jobs. I realized I don't need to travel to have that, so I have intentionally sought to create a life filled with things that matter to me. I've stepped away from this idea of being busy all the time and being productive all the time. It is okay to rest, it is okay to do nothing at all. It is okay to play. I can be ambitious without working 12 hours a day. I don't have to live that life. I don't have to chase the next thing or the newest this or that. I don't need to be a slave to debt. Chasing the American Dream is why so many people are worn out, depressed, exhausted and unhappy. I choose none of that. Sitting on the steps of the Cattedrale di Sant'Andrea in Amalfi, Italy eating gelato and watching the passeggiata. Seeing people greet and chat with each other, enjoying the presence of each other was a great experience. In suburban America, people go from their homes, sit in traffic to get to work, go back home and repeat day in and day out. To me, that is not life, that is the living dead. Being in Rio and experiencing a great sense of community made me realize how much I value friendship and community. Travel has helped me realize what I want and what I don't. I can live a life of joy, love and purpose whether I'm sitting in my living room or sitting in a cafe in Nairobi. Life is mine to make of it what I want, and it's okay to reject the status quo. It's important to do what makes my heart sing, whether other people understand it or not. This is how I maintain my mental health, choosing me and the things that matter to me daily and leaving behind the things that weigh me down. This is for me, the ultimate self-care.

What is your most therapeutic travel destination for stress relief and self-care?

I like destinations that offer a variety of options because therapeutic for me is having the option to go out and enjoy activities or to stay in and be pampered. A great view is essential as is having a body of water within walking distance. It would have to be the Amalfi Coast, Italy for the sea and amazing food and views. Other amazing places would be Nairobi and Mombasa (Kenya), Rio de Janeiro, Brazil. These are places that resonate with my spirit.

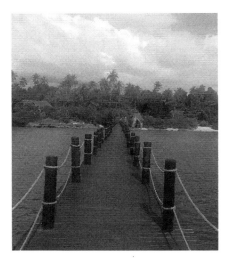

Whats is the most important items you have in your carryon and why?

My priority pass. Lounge access is essential. Helps me travel with comfort and allows me access to facilities such as showers and a space to relax

Favorite Calming Beverage or Food to consume while traveling and why?

Water. Especially when I'm in transit for 20 hours. Water is life.

Favorite Calming Music or Audio to listen to while traveling?

I still have an iPod shuffle, on it I have everything from Brazilian R&B to Australian rap music to Rock.

Favorite Keepsake that keeps you calm or grounded while traveling?

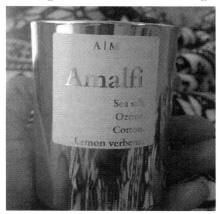

Tammy Freeman

What is your most hilarious travel memory?

On my 3rd visit to Rio, I stayed for 2 months. At the time, I didn't speak Portuguese but I would find great places to go all around Rio. I would just go places without a clue where I was. The issue this trip was getting back to where I stayed. While uber is rampant in Rio, if you're in a busy area and can't communicate where you are or understand what the driver is saying it becomes difficult. Long story short, I was somewhere in Rio and couldn't get home because I couldn't understand my Uber driver when he called me. I was out of the tourist area and no one spoke English (which I didn't expect them to anyway). I finally got a cab, the driver didn't speak English but somehow we were able to communicate. To top it off, I didn't have money for a cab since I expected to take an Uber. So I had to communicate to him to stop at a bank (and only a specific bank because some banks would charge a fee others would not), the first banks' ATM didn't work. It was a mess, but also funny. He was a good sport, we were both confused. I made it home and made a new acquaintance.

What is your most memorable or touching travel experience?

I have many, but the one that pops into my head was my experience in Cairo, Egypt. A man asked me where I was from and I told him the U.S., which he replied, "welcome home, Princess'. Now, that could have just been his standard pickup line LOL, but that was my first time on the continent of Africa so it was touching to hear the words, "welcome home".

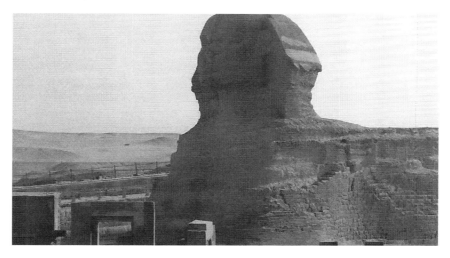

What is the worst travel experience you ever had?

Can't think of one.

Favorite Travel Hack?

I choose my destinations based on flight deals. Flights and accommodations are the most expensive items when traveling. I remain flexible and grab flight deals as opposed to being fixated on a specific place to go. Flight deals can be had to nearly anywhere, eventually, I'll make it to all the places I want to go to.

What is your travel Ritual for keeping calm and maintaining your inner zen?

Breathing, counting and grounding.

Best Travel Tip Advice?

Immersive travel experience can break you open, it can challenge the limits of what you've believed to be true in an amazing and even sometimes, heart-wrenching way. Let it.

Why is addressing mental health in and self-care with as it relates to people of color so important in the travel community?

> I think some people think of travel as a treat or as a reward after hard work. For me it is not. I deserve good things, period. I don't need to reward myself after I've toiled away at a job for 60 plus hours a week. Travel is part of my life, it is my "reward" for living. It is how I have new experiences and meet the world with the wonder of a child learning new things. It is how I challenge my reality, my views, it is how I break down barriers. It is often a mirror of myself and where I need to lean in, parts of me that need healing and attention through understanding, love and grace. Travel has broken me open in ways I can't describe and I'm so much better for it.

Although we travel often for our mental health, the topic is not emphasized due to shame and stigma. How can we normalize this conversation among the travel communities of color?

> Mental health in general needs to be normalized in our communities. I feel like there are lots of resources and the conversation is being had; however, there are still some pockets where mental health is stigmatized.

WEBSITE
www.soulandstoryinc.com

EMAIL
impact@soulandstoryinc.com

INSTAGRAM HANDLE
@soulandstoryinc

FACEBOOK PAGE
https://www.facebook.com/soulandstoryinc/

Travel Jokes

No one:

Me on my way to work: If I quit my job now I can be in Greece by 3pm

CHAPTER 41

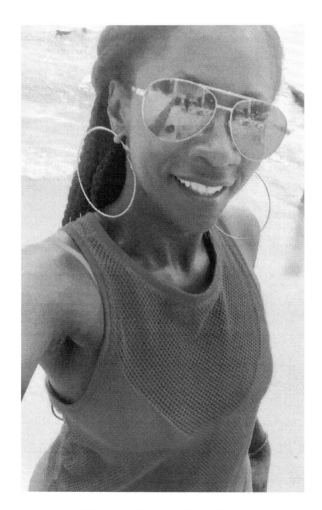

Kristin Riddle

World Travel Therapist

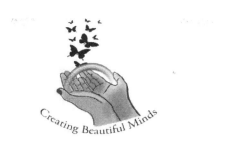

Travel Quote or Travel Mantra you live by
"Life will always be in session, whether you stay or whether you go!
Take the trip already, what are you waiting for?"

Travel Influencer/ Brand Summary
Angela L. Mull is a Licensed Marriage Family Therapist in Los Angeles. She serves a lot of clients who struggle with anxiety, depression and trauma-related issues. Her goal is to use other creative expressions whether that is art, music, dance, travel (exposure) and other evidence-based practices as an alternative to medication and talk therapy.

How has Traveling helped you maintain your mental health as it relates to self-care?
With balancing Motherhood/career I began to understand the importance of having an outlet or escape,travel I did not always present itself and I would have to often take virtual trips but closing my eyes imagining the places I wanted to be while taking a hot bubble bath whenever time permitted. Now as an Empty Nester I'm able to actually take those trips to places once imagined. Traveling has helped me temporarily escape the hustle of a demanding career serving others, it has helped me restore my energy physically by getting the adequate rest I would not otherwise get if I were home or at work, it has helped me recalibrate my mind by resting my thoughts and focusing on my inner self and not what's happening around me or with others, it has given me the mental space to think of more creative insight on ways to build my business, a greater sense of gratitude and appreciation for my life by seeing other cultures, scenery, and perspectives in the world it's made me more intentional of just living the best life for me.

What is your most therapeutic travel destination for stress relief and self-care?
The island of Wailea Maui, Hawaii

Whats is the most important items you have in your carryon and why?
3 things I keep in my carry on are earbuds/earplugs, snacks (nuts or protein bar) and toothpaste/brush. You never know when you will have a snoring seatmate or crying baby on your flight. Although we can empathetic to both we want to have a peaceful flight so popping those earbuds in is mandatory. I learned the hard way by having a flight delay on the tarmac to always have extra snacks on deck. Oh yeah, that toothbrush and toothpaste are necessary!God forbid you to get stuck or delayed on a flight and have that bad breath for hours or days yuck!! Nobody, even yourself wants to smell it after flying for hours Nothing worse for me with waking up with a bad

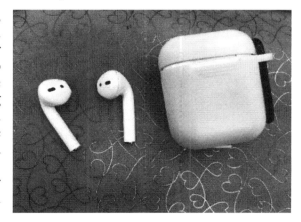

taste or bad breath. Especially if your Boo is waiting to pick you up at your final destination, stay ready! Xoxo

Favorite Calming Beverage or Food to consume while traveling and why?

Herbal non-caffeinated tea such as chamomile, ginger, and peppermint give me a calming yet refreshing feeling so that I'm able to relax and have the invigorating mental clarity I need to stay focused while traveling. I stay away from caffeine coffee, energy drinks and alcohol although they give me a false sense of alertness they seem to make me more anxious.

Favorite Calming Music or Audio to listen to while traveling?

I tend to opt for a variety of calming sounds/tunes while traveling. This could be smooth jazz, slow gospel, R&B music, meditative recordings, or a nice podcast. It just depends on the length of travel and #travelmood

Favorite Keepsake that keeps you calm or grounded while traveling?

Pictures of my children and grandchildren keep me grounded while traveling something about seeing those beautiful faces makes me feel accomplished and happy in my soul.

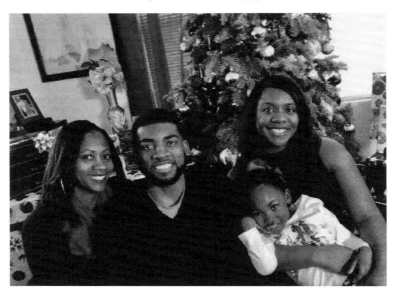

What is your most hilarious travel memory?

My most recent hilarious travel moment was while enjoying the waves on the beach in Oahu, I noticed something swimming next to me and it was a giant sea turtle! You should have seen me trying to run from it but the waves were so strong it was like I was in slow motion and I fell down, scraped my knee and the turtle calmly swam away in the other direction (hilarious) he wasn't even thinking about me LOL...

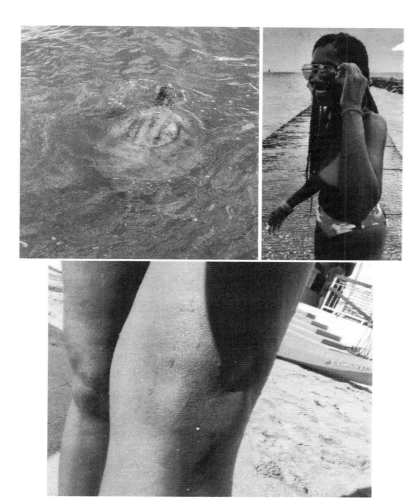

What is your most memorable or touching travel experience?

My most touching memories have always been meeting retirees at happy hour. Talking to them and listening to them share their stories (whether embellished or not LOL). I've learned a lot from them and have been given a lot of sound advice to apply to business, finance, marriage, child-rearing and life. What a joy to be able to retire and travel with both mental and physical health! #MyGoal

What is the worst travel experience you ever had?

My worst travel experience was one holiday my flight was delayed 3 hours, people were scattered all over airport terminals sleeping. We finally board the aircraft just to get stuck another 2 hours on the tarmac unable to take off! I was hungry and of course, it was the holiday so there were more restless children on the flights.

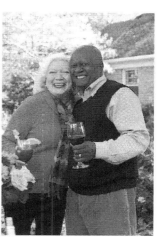

Favorite Travel Hack?

Find a low interest no annual fee credit card and rack up points and cash in on the incentives! This has helped me save hundreds, perhaps thousands of dollars on airfare, hotel and car rentals. I've been able to share this with my boyfriend and family so now we are planning on a big family trip that won't cost so much.

What is your travel Ritual for keeping calm and maintaining your inner zen?

I don't go out of the house on a daily without praying first! And this is definitely something I do even more while traveling, in the Uber, in the airport, and while in the air. Other things I've done is closing my eyes for a little guided meditation and deep controlled breathing in times of turbulence.

Best Travel Tip Advice?

Pre-pack early. Having those things that I know I can't live without packed early saves me from forgetting them. Get out early on travel day, this way your prepared to expect the unexpected and you won't feel the pressure or anxiety of the unexpected happening, you'll have that extra time to just breathe! Again "LIFE is ALWAYS in Session."

Why is addressing mental health in and self-care with as it relates to people of color so important in the travel community?

Many people of color have been conditioned to stay within "our communities" or comfort zones therefore many have not seen life outside of where they live. Sometimes these communities are afflicted with crime, violence, poverty or limited opportunities for growth and can cause Post Traumatic Stress Disorder (PTSD), anxiety and depression. Many don't realize why they have or experience these feelings because they've become desensitized to their surroundings. Being able to travel for self-care even for a short/brief period of time can alleviate some of these symptoms.

Although we travel often for our mental health, the topic is not emphasized due to shame and stigma. How can we normalize this conversation among the travel communities of color?

Great question! Having this book and other guides (articles, blogs, travel clubs etc) promoting mental health travel awareness is a good start to expressing the benefits of travel and mental health. As a clinician, I often encourage my clients to have self-care activities that include taking time to travel and explore whether it be taking a mini weekend trip or longer vacation. We spend a lot of time taking time working for a living to provide for our families or being competitive with societal norms we are often shamed or guilted for taking care of ourselves and for taking time off work being viewed as lazy or not motivated to do and have more. It is often said, "We have to work harder and need to always be striving to get ahead." Overextending ourselves and not taking time out for self-care can cause mental exhaustion which can lead to numerous psychological problems and addictive behaviors if we're not careful.

WEBSITE

AngelaMullTherapy.Com

EMAIL

angela@angelamulltherapy.com

INSTAGRAM HANDLE

@creatingbeautifulminds

FACEBOOK PAGE

Creating Beautiful Minds

Travel Jokes

  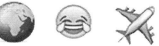

Popeye's Chicken Sandwich is for people that act fancy flying first class on Spirit.

CHAPTER 42

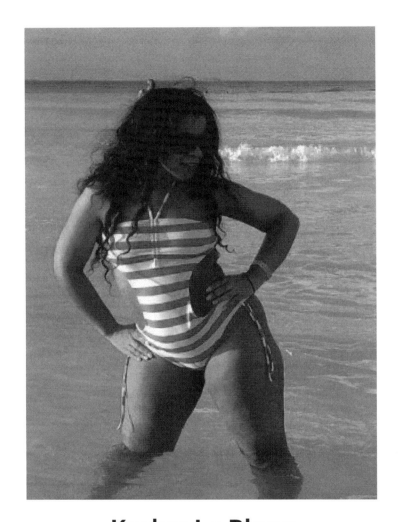

Karlyn Le Blanc
Black Girls Travel Therapy

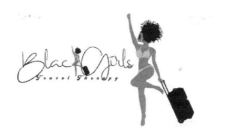

Travel Quote or Travel Mantra you live by
Traveling is Therapy, it promotes healing and happiness.

How has Traveling helped you maintain your mental health as it relates to self-care?
Traveling keeps me balanced and it's vital to my quality of life. It promotes happiness within, motivates me, and renews my creative side.

What is your most therapeutic travel destination for stress relief and self-care?
St. Lucia

Whats is the most important items you have in your carryon and why?
Swim Suits make me feel sexy, free and uninhibited. 2. Essential Oils heal my body, mind, and soul. 3. SunGlasses protect my eyes and make me feel cool.

Favorite Calming Beverage or Food to consume while traveling and why?
Ginger tea is my saving grace, it calms my spirit, gets rid of nausea and settles my stomach.

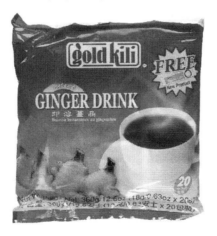

Favorite Calming Music or Audio to listen to while traveling?
I don't listen to anything when I travel.

Favorite Keepsake that keeps you calm or grounded while traveling?
Goddess waist beads

What is your most hilarious travel memory?
Playing in the hot mud in the Sulphur Springs Mud Bath in St. Lucia.

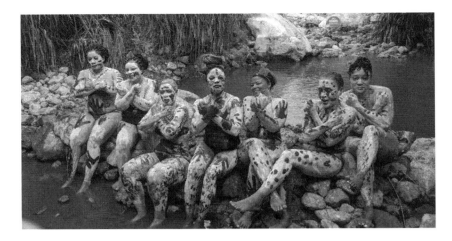

What is your most memorable or touching travel experience?

The most memorable travel experience was doing mission work with children in Jamaica.

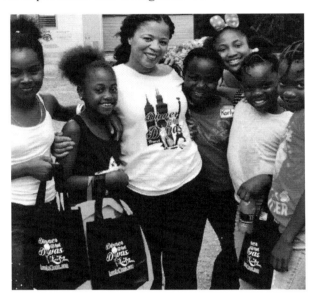

What is the worst travel experience you ever had?

Havana, Cuba was my worst travel experience. The language barrier and the travel band added to the negative experience. The people were rude and I felt totally disconnected.

Favorite Travel Hack?

I use my American Express Delta Rewards card for everything (bills, gas, food) to accumulate miles to travel for free. However, I pay it off every month.

What is your travel Ritual for keeping calm and maintaining your inner zen?

My travel ritual is having a nude moment wherever I go. It can be under the waterfalls, rainforest, beach, ocean, sauna, or balcony, being naked makes me feel liberated and powerful.

Karlyn Le Blanc

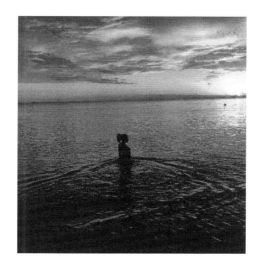

Best Travel Tip Advice?

    Its safer, cheaper, and more fun to travel with a group. You'll save on transportation from the airport to destination and and excursions

Why is addressing mental health in and self-care with as it relates to people of color so important in the travel community?

    People are dying every day from mental health issues, stress and depression being the main culprits. By educating our black communities we can save lives, by informing them that traveling is the cure. Traveling adds years to our lives and promotes happiness.

Although we travel often for our mental health, the topic is not emphasized due to shame and stigma. How can we normalize this conversation among the travel communities of color?

    More people need to speak out about their mental health issues and share how traveling helped. I suffered from severe depression for years and finally I decided to take my life back and live happily ever after. My key to happiness was traveling. I prescribe a trip every 3 months even if its a road trip.

WEBSITE
BlackGirlsTravelTherapy.com

EMAIL
blackgirlstraveltherapy@gmail.com

INSTAGRAM HANDLE
Black Girls Travel Therapy

FACEBOOK PAGE
Black Girls Travel Therapy

Travel Jokes

  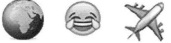

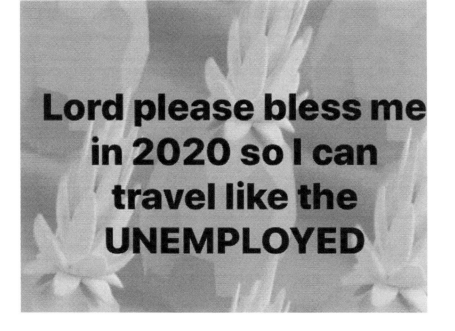

CHAPTER 43

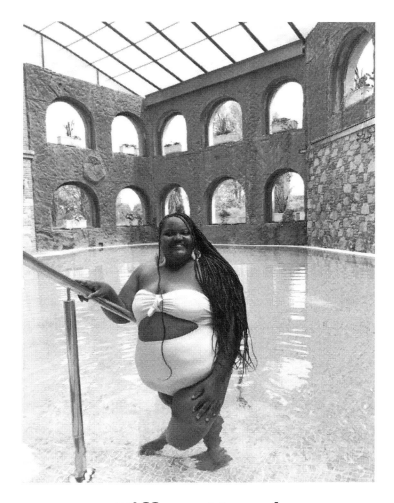

Tiffany Heard

Body Positive Travels

Travel Quote or Travel Mantra you live by
You only have one life to live so you live it well.
Living my best life one country at a time.

Travel Influencer/ Brand Summary
Sweet Tiffy's Inspirations was created to inspire others to travel the world. As it evolves my focus is now on helping women to increase self-esteem and confidence to accomplish goals that they want to achieve.

How has Traveling helped you maintain your mental health as it relates to self-care?
Working a 9-5 job in the Social Work field can cause stress as it is a profession where you are constantly caring for others. Taking a vacation allows you to mentally leave the stress behind. My vacations include the beach and something adventurous that I have never before.

What is your most therapeutic travel destination for stress relief and self-care?
My most therapeutic vacation was to Mexico City on a horse ranch called Las Ranchos Cascadas. It was very relaxing while there I was able to eat daily fresh food cooked by staff, ride horses, massages, hot tubs, and waterfalls. During the time they had several writer retreats.

Whats is the most important items you have in your carryon and why?
Clothes- underwear, leggings, T-shirt- My checked-in luggage has been lost before Snacks, Medication Charger Phone, Ipad Book or Magazine Passport Credit cards

Favorite Calming Beverage or Food to consume while traveling and why?
I love to go on food tours and take cooking classes when I travel. Learning how to cook local food is an important part of immersing myself in the culture.

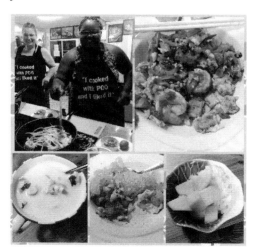

Favorite Calming Music or Audio to listen to while traveling?

I love listening to Gospel music on Pandora

Favorite Keepsake that keeps you calm or grounded while traveling?

I don't have a particular keepsake but my mom keeps me grounded by checking in with her nightly so she makes sure that I am safe.

What is your most hilarious travel memory?

Most hilarious Moment: My cousin was laughing and teasing me for being afraid of the elephants ! The elephant guide said to be careful because they like to roll around in the water. 15 min later I hear my cousin screaming. The elephant went backward and so did she! Thank God she knows how to swim.. the joke was on her.

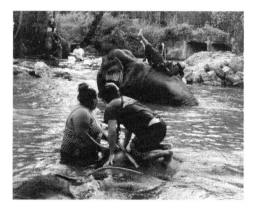

What is your most memorable or touching travel experience?

Going to Ghana to volunteer at school and me and this little girl bonding instantly over coca-cola

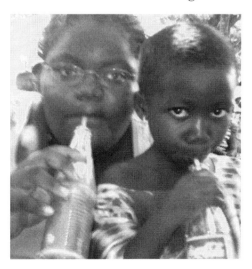

What is the worst travel experience you ever had?

Traveling to Ghana for the first time, my bag from LA to San Francisco and they gave me a box to put all my belongings. Once we arrived in Germany our flight was delayed. Once we arrived in Ghana we did not have luggage for 3 days.

Favorite Travel Hack?

> Using accommodation sites such as Airbnb and the hostel world to find cheap accommodations. Saving money on the Digit App. Using the Chase Credit Card reserve for flight points.

What is your travel Ritual for keeping calm and maintaining your inner zen?

> I don't have a specific ritual that keeps me calm. But I make sure on every trip I do something that gets me out of my comfort zone, hang out with the locals, find a beach or pool, experience the food.

Best Travel Tip Advice?

> Take a solo trip. Life is to short to wait on others. Many people will persuade you not to go because they feel it's not safe but go anyway. Send them a postcard and say how much you missed them. Lol Yes, it is scary but it will be exciting, liberating, learning process and you will meet som many new people along the way.

Why is addressing mental health in and self-care with as it relates to people of color so important in the travel community?

> It super important because people of color tend to carry the weight of burdens on their shoulders. Especially women of color often care for spouses, kids, family and work while neglecting themselves in the process. We need to encourage the thought of taking the following types of vacation: solo, girls, friend or baecation as a form of self-care. Travel can include staycation, domestic or international travel.

Although we travel often for our mental health, the topic is not emphasized due to shame and stigma. How can we normalize this conversation among the travel communities of color?

> I think that we can normalize this by having conversations, conferences, retreats, churches to address mental health concerns and solutions such as therapy to deal with people dealing with mental health. We should also normalize therapy and not call people crazy because they need to seek help.

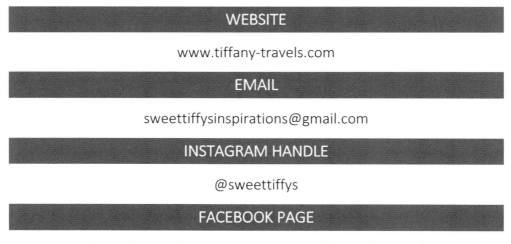

WEBSITE

www.tiffany-travels.com

EMAIL

sweettiffysinspirations@gmail.com

INSTAGRAM HANDLE

@sweettiffys

FACEBOOK PAGE

https://www.facebook.com/sweettiffysinspirations/

Travel Jokes

  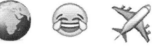

When your plane lands & the person next to you starts clapping

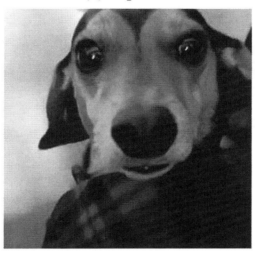

CHAPTER 44

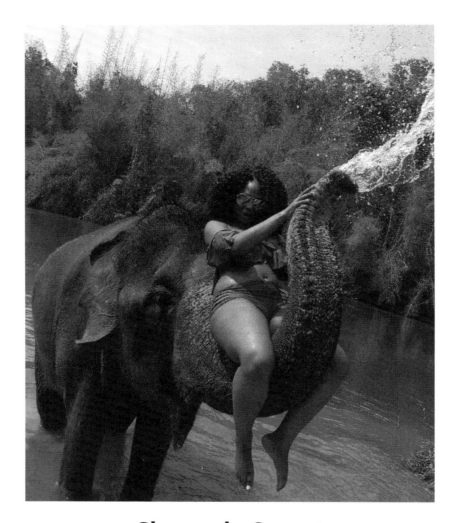

Shanayla Sweat

Time Traveler

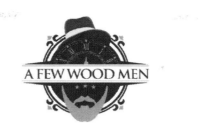

Travel Quote or Travel Mantra you live by
Travel while you can, because you won't be able to travel forever.

Travel Influencer/ Brand Summary
A Few Wood Men's desire is that your wooden watch brings to remembrance the character, resilience, kingship, and honor of that special man of distinction.

How has Traveling helped you maintain your mental health as it relates to self-care?
Traveling is a huge part of my self-care regimen. Anytime that I feel unfocused, distracted, ungrateful, or uninspired I travel and my eyes are opened up to the world around me. Traveling keeps me grounded and allows me to clear my mind when it's unsettled.

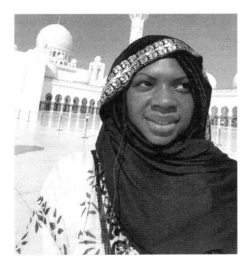

What is your most therapeutic travel destination for stress relief and self-care?
So far my most therapeutic travel destination has been to Thailand. While in Thailand, I was constantly reminded of all the things that I have been blessed with and able to accomplish. The best stress relievers while there, was bathing elephants and taking advantage of some of the best full-body massages.

Whats is the most important items you have in your carryon and why?
The most important item to take in your carryon is bug spray. Bug spray has saved my life in so many countries!

Favorite Calming Beverage or Food to consume while traveling and why?
I am a hot wing connoisseur and love to try wings in every country that I travel to! It reminds me of home and opens my taste buds to new flavors.

The Ultimate Self-Care Guide for Travelers of Color

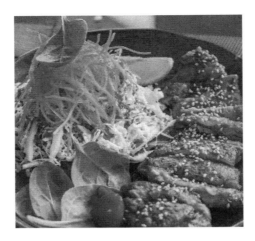

Favorite Calming Music or Audio to listen to while traveling?

I always tune into a Big Sean album when I am traveling.

Favorite Keepsake that keeps you calm or grounded while traveling?

I actually don't have a favorite keepsake that I take with me on trips.

What is your most hilarious travel memory?

My most hilarious moment probably came out of South Africa! My travel buddy and I went to a township party, where it went down! Drinking, dancing, partying, cops...I'll stops there lol.

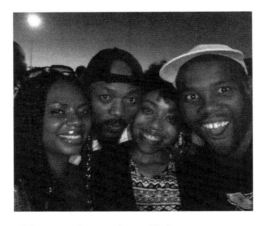

my journal on my trips and watching movies on long flights.

What is your most memorable or touching travel experience?

My most memorable experience to date would have to be going through the safaris in South Africa. We were so close to the animals. It absolutely blew my mind seeing their true beauty!

What is the worst travel experience you ever had?

The worse travel experience that I had was probably in Paris, France. I was not impressed with the food, I had tours scheduled unexpectedly canceled, a shocking reveal of the Mona Lisa...it was not a great experience.

Favorite Travel Hack?

My favorite travel hack would have to be getting travel deals on flights through The Travel Deal.

Shanayla Sweat

What is your travel Ritual for keeping calm and maintaining your inner zen?

My travel ritual would have to be writing in

Best Travel Tip Advice?

My best travel advice would be to have an open mind and always plan for a plan B. Things don't always go as planned or as expected and you don't have as much control being on a trip, so the best advice would be to be open to all types of scenarios and experiences.

Why is addressing mental health in and self-care with as it relates to people of color so important in the travel community?

Mental Health is so important to not only the travel community but to our community and village as people of African descent. Traveling allows us to conquer our fears, restore our confidence, and expose us to new levels. It's important to showcase travel as an avenue to relieve stress while building our spirit and cultivating our minds.

Although we travel often for our mental health, the topic is not emphasized due to shame and stigma. How can we normalize this conversation among the travel communities of color?

I think we could normalize the conversation by emphasizing activities that we participate in for self-care while on travel. If we are going to the spa, journaling, or meditating those are things that we can highlight and discuss when sharing our travel experiences. We can also be more transparent about our mental health struggles and ways that we are managing them. I try to be transparent with my journey by sharing with others my journey with therapy.

WEBSITE

www.afewwoodmen.com

EMAIL

info@afewwoodmen.com

INSTAGRAM HANDLE

www.instagram.com/afewwoodmen_

FACEBOOK PAGE

facebook.com/AfewWoodMen

Travel Jokes

THERE SHOULD BE SYMPATHY CARDS FOR HAVING TO GO BACK TO WORK AFTER VACATION.

CHAPTER 45

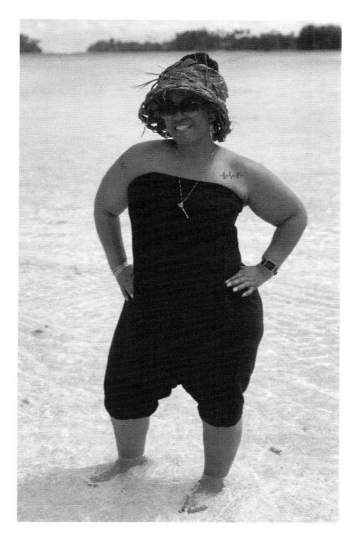

Adrienne Ferguson

Travel Quote or Travel Mantra you live by
"You only have one life to live & if you're always living in fear, you're going to miss out on a lot!"

How has Traveling helped you maintain your mental health as it relates to self-care?

Traveling snaps me out of negative energy, depression, and stress. It's is a way for me to heal my soul, to cleanse my mind, and open my heart. Being in a different environment and around different cultures is very therapeutic for my mind. It takes me out of my comfort zone and forces me to focus on what's happening at the moment instead of what happened in the past. After I'm away, I return home with new awareness and fresh perspectives, ready to take on life's challenges and opportunities again.

What is your most therapeutic travel destination for stress relief and self-care?

This is going to sound funny but Universal Studios and Disneyland in Los Angeles, CA. When I'm there, I turn into a kid again and all of my troubles fade away...I love to laugh, have fun and enjoy all of the characters/Rides.

Whats is the most important items you have in your carryon and why?

The most important items in my carryon are my Laptop, Beats Headphones, Thumb Drive and my Travel Pillow & Blanket. I use my headphones to watch the movies on the plane but if by some chance the plane doesn't offer that, I have over 100 movies on my Thumb Drive and I can watch them on my Laptop. Not all airlines have blankets and pillows, so I also have my own.

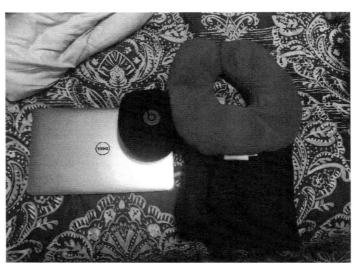

Favorite Calming Beverage or Food to consume while traveling and why?

My favorite calming beverage and food when I'm traveling is coffee with Bailey's Irish Cream and Biscoff Cookies.

Adrienne Ferguson

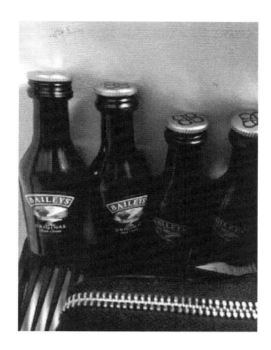

Favorite Calming Music or Audio to listen to while traveling?

I have a mix of 80's, 90's and early 2000's R&B music that I always listen to when traveling.

Favorite Keepsake that keeps you calm or grounded while traveling?

I don't really have a keepsake but communicating with my mother every chance I get helps to keep me calm and grounded.

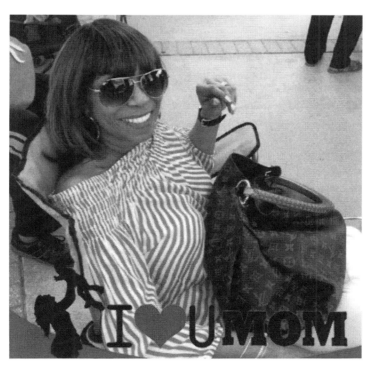

What is your most hilarious travel memory?.?

My most hilarious travel memory was when I was trying to conquer my fear of snakes in Sydney. My brother held it first, so I said I was going to hold it next, BUT only with the Zoo Keeper...I'm not ready to hold it on my own yet. Everything went really well UNTIL he started to move...That's when I lost it. HAHA

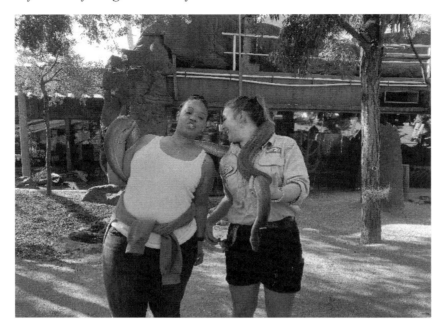

What is your most memorable or touching travel experience?

My most memorable or touching travel experience was when I was in Cuba. That country and the people really gave me a different outlook on life. It made me appreciate everything that I have and not worry about the things I don't. They don't have a lot at all but you would never know it...They appreciate what they have every day and never complain.

What is the worst travel experience you ever had?

The worst travel experience I've ever had was traveling to Turks and Caicos Island and American Airlines losing all of my luggage and it was never recovered. Not only was it never recovered, but they also gave me the hardest time about reimbursing me for my items...I kept questioning why I packed what I did and didn't believe some of my items listed. I had to buy everything I needed from the island and it wasn't cheap...But the Island and the people are beautiful.

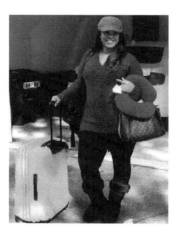

Favorite Travel Hack?

I wear compression socks so my ankles don't swell

What is your travel Ritual for keeping calm and maintaining your inner zen?

Before I travel anywhere, I pray before I leave my destination...Every Single Time.

Best Travel Tip Advice?

Take lots of pictures, get out and explore, meet the locals, try their food and try to learn their culture. Go on excursions, try to do things spur of the moment (don't plan everything). Learn a few words of the language in every country you visit and leave space in your bag to bring back memories. ALSO, carry your passport with you EVERYWHERE!!!

Why is addressing mental health in and self-care with as it relates to people of color so important in the travel community?

Addressing mental health is important because, in the African American community, many misunderstand what mental health is. Many believe that a mental health condition is a personal weakness and are reluctant to discuss it and/or seek treatment because of the shame and stigma associated with such conditions.

Although we travel often for our mental health, the topic is not emphasized due to shame and stigma. How can we normalize this conversation among the travel communities of color?

Talk about it more and stop making it seem like it's something to be ashamed of.

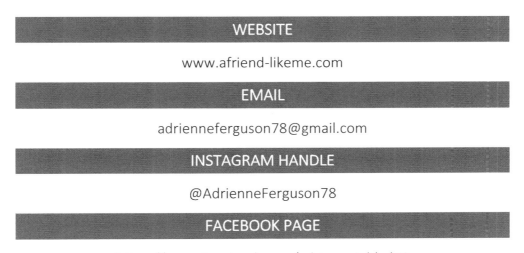

WEBSITE
www.afriend-likeme.com

EMAIL
adrienneferguson78@gmail.com

INSTAGRAM HANDLE
@AdrienneFerguson78

FACEBOOK PAGE
https://www.facebook.com/adriennejahkel78

Travel Jokes

The airport is a lawless place. 7am? Drink a beer. Tired? Sleep on the floor. Hungry? Chips now cost $17

CHAPTER 46

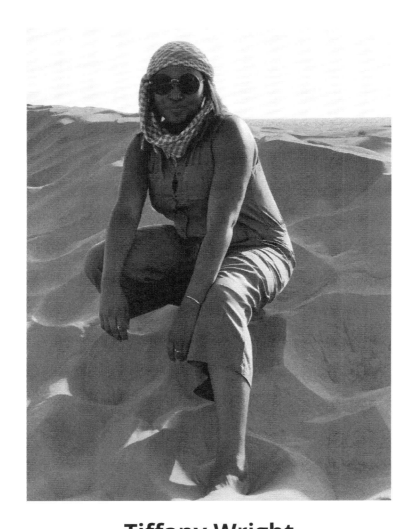

Tiffany Wright

Traveling Empowerment Brunches

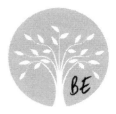

Travel Quote or Travel Mantra you live by
"Not all those who wander are lost." – J.R.R. Tolkien

Travel Influencer/ Brand Summary

My brand is centered on promoting empowerment and transformational messages of self-love wellness to women through brunches that take place all around the world. This is expressed through my non-profit Coco Coalition, where I curate healing events for Black women around the world, my platform The BE Life where I provide resources and tools that promote self-love and mental health awareness, and my profession as a mental health clinician.

How has Traveling helped you maintain your mental health as it relates to self-care?

I have tapped into creating experiences of awe and have come to know that awe is essential to me experiencing a deep connection to myself and God. In travel, I experience awe mainly through natural landscapes, but also experience it through observing different ways of living. I have found that many other nations care for people very differently than the US, therefore, my mind also gets a chance to slow down, be present, and release focus on productivity. Going places that I can sit in wonderment allows me to focus on the positive, be mindful of my stress level, and just play, explore or relax.

What is your most therapeutic travel destination for stress relief and self-care?

I don't have a "go-to" however I would say Bali has been an extremely therapeutic destination due to how intricate spirituality is to their lives, as well as the serenity the water, flora, and plants provide. It also helps that you can get really inexpensive massages!

Whats is the most important items you have in your carryon and why?

Well, I am a team carryon so I typically have everything that I will be traveling with. My clothes, shoes, undergarments, basic toiletries, first aid kit to always include Benadryl, bug repellant, my camera, extra portable chargers, my journal, towel, washcloth, hair scarf, accessories, and travel documents.

Favorite Calming Beverage or Food to consume while traveling and why?

I typically pack an assortment of herbal teas to bring on travels, and always have a stress relief or lavender tea. My favorite brand is traditional medicinals. For long flights, I bring protein shakes and bars, so I can have if I get hungry.

Favorite Calming Music or Audio to listen to while traveling?

I have a classical playlist, as well as John Coltrane.

Favorite Keepsake that keeps you calm or grounded while traveling?

I never travel without my journal. There's always an opportunity for reflection.

What is your most hilarious travel memory?

In Durban, people kept assuming I was Zulu to the extent that when I told a local I wasn't, she kept asking if I was lying, and believed I faked my US accent.

What is your most memorable or touching travel experience?

When I was in Johannesburg, I hosted a women's empowerment brunch and was able to collect funds and donations for tampons, which I then gathered and delivered (with the help of a local) to a high school in Alexandra for girls. It was such an amazing experience.

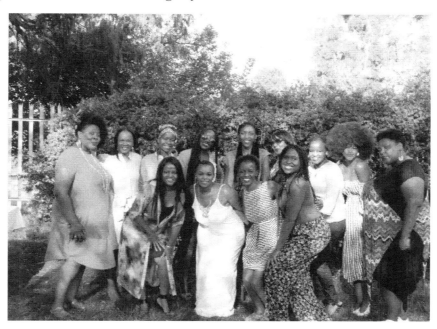

What is the worst travel experience you ever had?

I can't necessarily re-call because I believe that in general there are challenges to almost any travel experience but it doesn't take away from the whole experience. In Bali, I got bit by red ants and had an allergic reaction towards the end of the trip. I couldn't wait to get home to take Benadryl because the bites were starting to become unbearable to the point of not being able to sleep.

Favorite Travel Hack?

To me, using Airbnb so I can get local recommendations, as well as grocery shops, in order to save a little money by cooking.

What is your travel Ritual for keeping calm and maintaining your inner zen?

Journaling and traveling with my Chinese Herbs for anxiety.

Best Travel Tip Advice?

Don't over plan 2. Go where locals go 3. Pack light 4. Be open "off the beaten path" experiences 5. Get travel insurance

Why is addressing mental health in and self-care with as it relates to people of color so important in the travel community?

Communities of color tend to ignore conversations about mental health and the necessities of self-care. We traditionally have "word-hard" mentalities, as well as "just keep going and be strong" approaches to life's challenges. Chronic stress continues to threaten our quality of life. Travel and self-care can be used as a means for de-stressing if done with intention. It's important to note that people are getting in debt because of travel or even using travel to fill voids, and garner validation and acknowledgment from others, and these are ways that travel and actually contribute to poor mental health. When people feel lost or sad, and want to travel, it can be dangerous, as being in such a vulnerable psychological state could lead to unsafe or impulsive behaviors while traveling. It's also important because if traveling alone, having a mental breakdown can be extremely dangerous and debilitating. Self-care is meant to rejuvenate, restore, and replenish...if travel even gets to a point that it causes more stress, it is not a helpful self-care tool. Addressing mental health with the travel community can also open dialogue about various types of travel such as that for transformative purposes, which can often be found with various retreats.

Although we travel often for our mental health, the topic is not emphasized due to shame and stigma. How can we normalize this conversation among the travel communities of color?

The more that travelers discuss their intentions, or psychological takeaways from trips, as opposed to just sharing their photos, the more normalized the conversation becomes. If individuals share more narratives around their emotional states before and during a trip, as well as any epiphanies experienced, these can become more common conversations. I often share information about my travels through the lens of mental health and personal development, therefore, its with the intention of showing people the connection between both. Now when I go on a trip, people anticipate the lessons I am going to share with them, that I experienced.

WEBSITE

www.livethebelife.com

EMAIL

beyou@livethebelife.com

INSTAGRAM HANDLE

tiffinspires

FACEBOOK PAGE

https://www.facebook.com/BlackBeautifulBrunch/

Travel Jokes

Running to the gate is my cardio.

CHAPTER 47

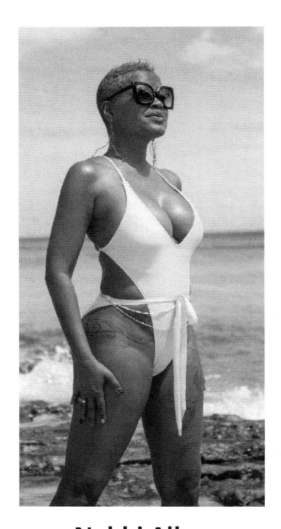

Nykki Allen

Luxury Travel Swimwear

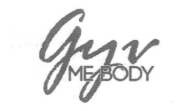

Travel Quote or Travel Mantra you live by
Travel is not a want; it's a NEED for me.

Travel Influencer / Brand Summary
My brand of swimwear focuses on luxury travel for Women and some Men's items. Our Allen Empire Page encourages couples to getaway, see the world and enjoy life. Both pages are travelers influenced.

How has Traveling helped you maintain your mental health as it relates to self-care?
WOW! Working in fashion for almost 3 decades, is sometimes VERY stressful, extremely fast-paced and your creative mind finds it difficult to rest. The ONLY time, I can realistically break away from that is when I'm on vacation. I can literally unplug, which is a NEED for me.

What is your most therapeutic travel destination for stress relief and self-care?
Barbados hands down.... it feels like the home I should live in daily.

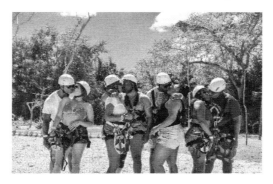

Whats is the most important items you have in your carryon and why?
I'm excellent at packing. I can pack at least 5 days of clothes, shoes and toiletries in a carryon just in case my luggage gets lost I can still have a change of clothes for a few days.

Favorite Calming Beverage or Food to consume while traveling and why?
Wine. Wine is my fave in any place. It calms my nerves.

Favorite Calming Music or Audio to listen to while traveling?
Nothing. I'm usually sleeping.

Favorite Keepsake that keeps you calm or grounded while traveling?
I never travel without my pillow. It's a comfort for me.

What is your most hilarious travel memory?

I get motion sickness. I was so sick on the catamaran, that I laid down. One of the staff took a pic with a bottle next to me.... lies. It was the motion sickness, but I have little proof.

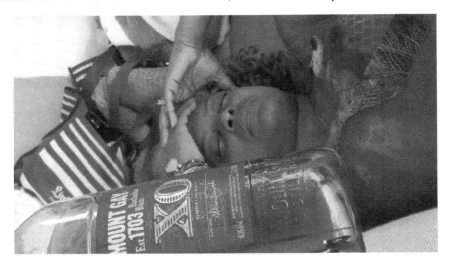

What is your most memorable or touching travel experience?

My husband and I renewed our 3rd year vow in Barbados with 2 other couples. Hands down, it was perfect.

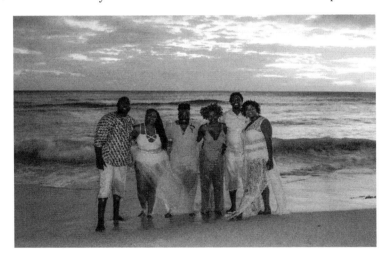

What is the worst travel experience you ever had?

Dominican in 2018. It wasn't horrible. It just wasn't great. #1 You have to know the people you can travel with. #2 the DR was just ok. There was nothing GREAT about it

Favorite Travel Hack?

Expedia or Priceline

What is your travel Ritual for keeping calm and maintaining your inner zen?

Spending plenty of time listening to and near the ocean. It's hypnotic for me. I like going to listen to it very early in the morning and late at night.

Nykki Allen

Best Travel Tip Advice?

If it's a long flight, fly business or first class if you can. No one likes sitting uncomfortably for 8 or more hours. Your body will thank you later.

Why is addressing mental health in and self-care with as it relates to people of color so important in the travel community?

Black and Brown people don't travel as much as they should. They think that they can START to travel after the kids grow up or after they retire or after this or that is paid off. The truth of the matter is that there are no guarantees that one will live to see all of those things come into fruition. Secondly, your children will learn to travel and enjoy life if they see you do it first. Thirdly balance is vital to living. Without it, we burn out and we're good no one including ourselves.

Although we travel often for our mental health, the topic is not emphasized due to shame and stigma. How can we normalize this conversation among the travel communities of color?

We posed a question at one of our Couples Staycations... If you could go anywhere in the world, where would you go and why? The couples got so involved in the answers by participation that a few of them are living those desires out in the next upcoming year. We have to make the topic, fun, interactive and enjoyable in order for people to feel safe talking about it.

WEBSITE

https://gyvmebody.net/

EMAIL

NYKIK@MSN.COM

INSTAGRAM HANDLE

Gyvmebody

Travel Jokes

I am:

- Single
- Taken
- ● At the airport

Looking For:

- A Man
- A Woman
- ● Someone to convince me that 5am is too early for wine

CHAPTER 48

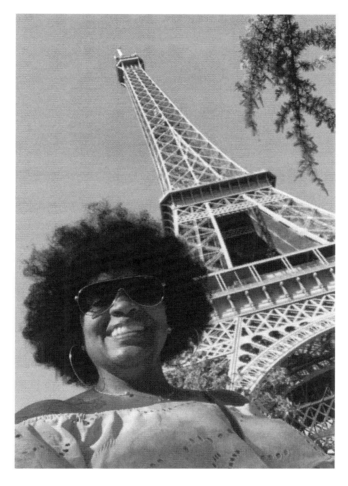

Yvette Christopher

*The Wild Adventures of Maddy's Traveling Granny
& Your Favorite Rich Auntie*

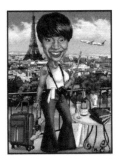

Maddy's Granny & Your Favorite Rich Auntie

Travel Quote or Travel Mantra you live by
Let's live our dreams, trip and fall a few times.

Travel Influencer / Brand Summary

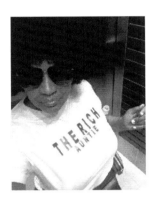

Yvette Christopher a retired lieutenant from the L.A County Sherriff's department. She became an instant social media phenom by posting her hilarious adventures of her and her beautiful granddaughter Maddy, heartfelt inspirational quotes, lavish restaurant and cocktails reviews and 10K Runners Medal chasing around the world. Loved by many the world could clearly see this was not your average grandma! At the age of 55, She was quickly coined the name "Maddy's Granny & Your Favorite Rich Auntie" was created by just living her life to the fullest and inspiring others to do the same no matter what age.

How has Traveling helped you maintain your mental health as it relates to self-care?

Traveling opens my mind to new things, adventure and uninhibited laughter and fun. It's incredible what a change of season does for the soul.

What is your most therapeutic travel destination for stress relief and self-care?

Paris, New York

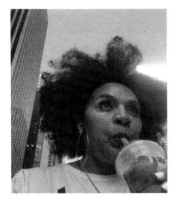

Whats is the most important items you have in your carryon and why?

Toothbrush and paste, wipes, hand sanitizer and deodorant, 1 pr of panties and phone charger. If there is an issue with the plane /airport, I can freshen up and call home.

Yvette Christopher

Favorite Calming Beverage or Food to consume while traveling and why?

Champagne / sparkling wine.

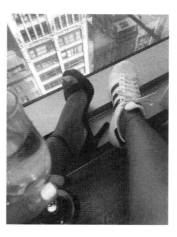

Favorite Calming Music or Audio to listen to while traveling?

Jazz, old school r & b, Luther, Anita

Favorite Keepsake that keeps you calm or grounded while traveling?

Pics of my family.

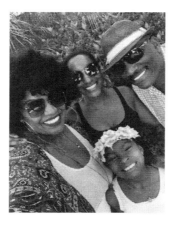

What is your most hilarious travel memory?

Pretending I was the tour guide in Paris and having everyone believe me.

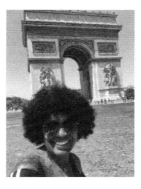

What is your most memorable or touching travel experience?

> Going to NY praying to get into the Wendy Williams show with no ticket. I received the last ticket. I gave her a gift, which she wears often. A bracelet that says, "How you doing?"

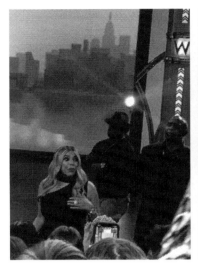 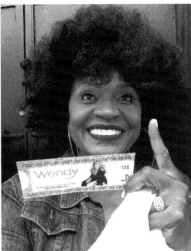

What is the worst travel experience you ever had?

> I've not had one. Thank God

Favorite Travel Hack?

> Safety gadgets for solo travelers

What is your travel Ritual for keeping calm and maintaining your inner zen?

> Prayer. I pray allll the time.

Best Travel Tip Advice?

> Don't be afraid to go alone. Plan ahead, research, go on a tour and pay in advance. Do all the things you like. Download a money conversion calculator and translator app. Learn a few words and phrases. Talk to the locals. Be brave.

Why is addressing mental health in and self-care with as it relates to people of color so important in the travel community?

> It's an important Period. So many ppl are not getting help for a multitude of reasons and it affects every aspect of their lives. Those really effected are a lot thinking of travel.

Although we travel often for our mental health, the topic is not emphasized due to shame and stigma. How can we normalize this conversation among the travel communities of color?

> Open honest dialogue and share personal stories. Offer help/assistance solutions.

Yvette Christopher

EMAIL

smalltown_grl17@yahoo.com

INSTAGRAM HANDLE

Sistaah

FACEBOOK PAGE

Yvette Harper Christopher

Maddys Grandma & Your Richh Auntie

Travel Jokes

Shout out to the guy making announcements at my gate. He said, and I quote, "Now boarding group A as in applebottom jeans and group B as in boots with the fur."

CHAPTER 49

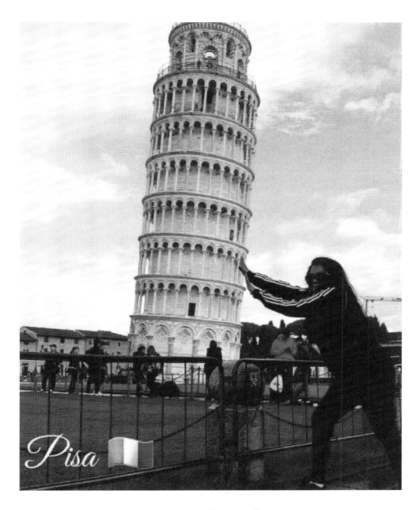

Lorena Garduno

Woman Owned Traveling Cigar Company

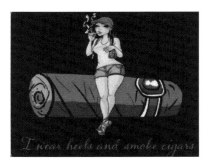

Travel Quote or Travel Mantra you live by

Pieces of life can be found through a cigar and traveling

Travel Influencer/ Brand Summary

A Traveling Latina owned Cigar Bar. What started out as a hobby and vice for relaxation turned a dream into reality. Facing the odds of a male-dominated industry, showing the world how my two passions cigars and travel have created room for me to live the life while influencing others to live out their dreams

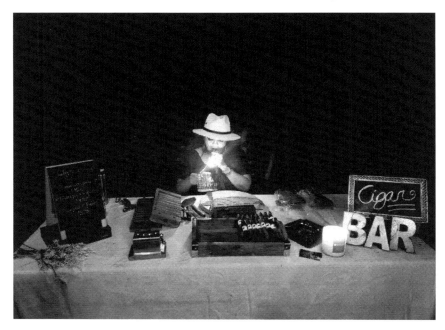

How has Traveling helped you maintain your mental health as it relates to self-care?

Traveling is my reset button. Needed to maintain my sanity. Traveling has helps me to put things into perspective. It is no longer a luxury. It is a necessity

What is your most therapeutic travel destination for stress relief and self-care?

Anywhere there is an ocean, sand, breeze

Whats is the most important items you have in your carryon and why?

Heartburn medication

Favorite Calming Beverage or Food to consume while traveling and why?

Chocolate

Lorena Garduno

Favorite Calming Music or Audio to listen to while traveling?

    Jazz Music

Favorite Keepsake that keeps you calm or grounded while traveling?

    Picture of my children

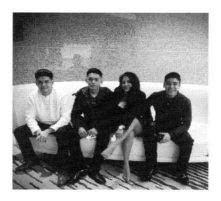

What is your most hilarious travel memory?

    Venice Italy Went during a flood

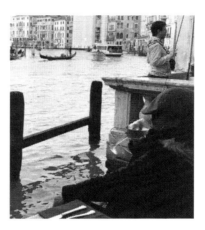

What is your most memorable or touching travel experience?

    Santorini Greece

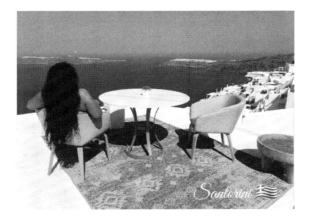

What is the worst travel experience you ever had?

> None yet Thank God!

Favorite Travel Hack?

> Can think of one at this moment

What is your travel Ritual for keeping calm and maintaining your inner zen.?

> Glass of wine and cigar prior to traveling

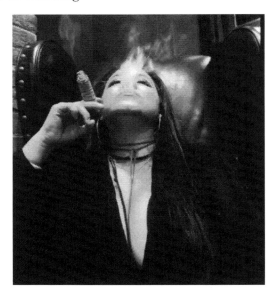

Best Travel Tip Advice?

> Be alert of your surrounding in a foreign country

Why is addressing mental health in and self-care with as it relates to people of color so important in the travel community?

> Traveling breaks that routine in any community. I like to call it self care, reset button. Life from a different perspective.

Although we travel often for our mental health, the topic is not emphasized due to shame and stigma. How can we normalize this conversation among the travel communities of color?

> I think this has nothing to do with color. Traveling has no color lines. Mental health does not discriminate. We all feel and experience the same.

Lorena Garduno

Travel Jokes

There are 3 types of people at the airport:
1. Get there early just so they can drink at the bar
2. Arrive 4 hours early and plant themselves at the gate in case the plane takes off ahead of schedule
3. Running to get to the gate 30 seconds before it closes

CHAPTER 50

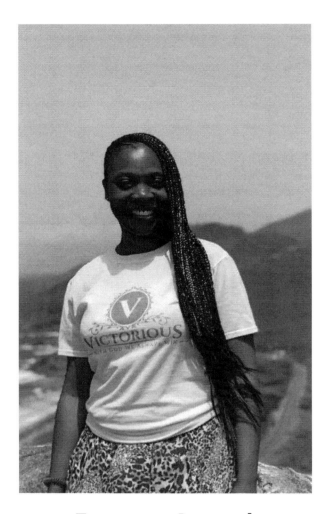

Frances Armad

Traveling Missionary with Style

Frances Armad

Travel Quote or Travel Mantra you live by
Traveling allows you to see God's entire creation

Travel Influencer/ Brand Summary

Modestly Awkward is a Podcast that shows people they can be themselves. As a fashion industry expert, I want to show women they don't have to show it all. They too can travel the world and be modest like me and still be chic and yet comfortable.

How has Traveling helped you maintain your mental health as it relates to self-care?

I have always enjoyed traveling. I travel as a Missionary and for leisure. When my grandmother passed away last year, I saw myself traveling more to clear my mind. Traveling has helped me to be able to heal. I cried as long and as many times I wanted. I was able to focus my attention on my environment and help escape some of my worries. When I arrived home, I felt better and was not in emotional pain. I will not say it is easy but traveling this year has helped. I went on Missionary trips as well as personal trips.

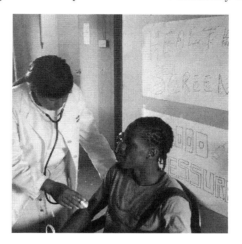

What is your most therapeutic travel destination for stress relief and self-care?

Most Therapeutic travel destinations would be London. I go with my friends every year and we like to do a tour to visit other countries. I enjoy the laughter, the shopping and also resting. We spent a day in Morocco for one year just shopping at the local flea market and talking with the natives.

Whats is the most important items you have in your carryon and why?

Bible

Favorite Calming Beverage or Food to consume while traveling and why?

Ginger Tea

Favorite Calming Music or Audio to listen to while traveling?

Gospel music

Favorite Keepsake that keeps you calm or grounded while traveling?

I have jewelry that my grandmother gave me. However, I keep those at home because I don't want to lose them

What is your most hilarious travel memory?

    I can't narrow it down to just one all of my trips are filled with smiles and laughter

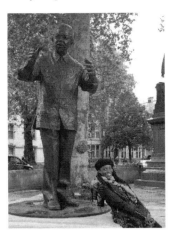

What is your most memorable or touching travel experience?

    Every trip is memorable!

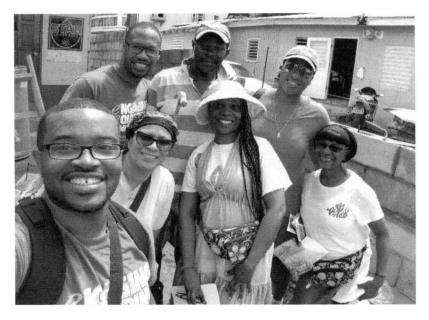

What is the worst travel experience you ever had?

    Jamaica, when I watched a guy in a motorcycle, snatched my friend'sE chain in broad daylight.

Favorite Travel Hack?

    I place all my clothes in ziplock bags for space and place. I like my suitcase to be very organized for easy access. I also buy a different suitcase each year

What is your travel Ritual for keeping calm and maintaining your inner zen?

    Pray and Singing while packing

Frances Armad

Best Travel Tip Advice?

ake every trip as an adventure. No expectations...

Why is addressing mental health in and self-care with as it relates to people of co or so important in the travel community?

Some places will not welcome people of color. You have to know who you are, be comfortable in your own skin.

Although we travel often for our mental health, the topic is not emphasized due to shame and stigma. How can we normalize this conversation among the travel communities of color?

Talk about fear of traveling, create a community that addresses some traveling concerns and updates.

EMAIL

frankeyume@gmail.com

INSTAGRAM HANDLE

modestly_awkward_podcast

FACEBOOK PAGE

Modestly Awkward

Travel Jokes

Imagine falling in love with someone and then finding out they clap their hands when the plane lands.

CHAPTER 51

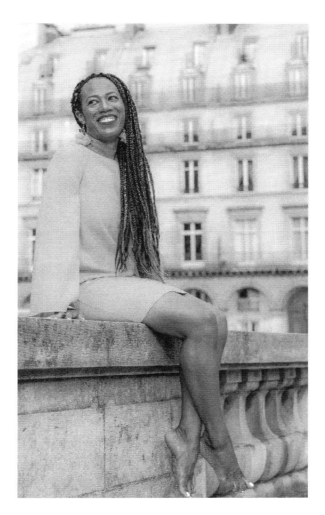

Roshida Dowe

Adult Gap Year

Travel Quote or Travel Mantra you live by
Taking a year off to travel can change your life.

Travel Influencer/ Brand Summary

Providing adult gap year guidance for those suffering from burnout or yearning to transform an element of their daily lives.

How has Traveling helped you maintain your mental health as it relates to self-care?

Traveling helps me gain space and distance from my everyday life. This space helps me see the things that are working and not working and allows me to make the changes necessary to live my best life.

What is your most therapeutic travel destination for stress relief and self-care?

Ohannesburg

Whats is the most important items you have in your carryon and why?

Eye mask and noise-canceling headphones for the best sleep on flights.

Favorite Calming Beverage or Food to consume while traveling and why?

Dark chocolate

Favorite Calming Music or Audio to listen to while traveling

I listen to a variety of podcasts while traveling.

Favorite Keepsake that keeps you calm or grounded while traveling?

I don't take keepsakes with me, but I pick up jewelry along the way.

What is your travel Ritual for keeping calm and maintaining your inner zen?

When flying, I don't go to the gate until right before boarding. The pre-boarding anxious energy from other travelers makes me anxious, so I avoid it.

Best Travel Tip Advice?

For last-minute trips, use Skyscanner's "Everywhere" feature to find the cheapest flights.

Why is addressing mental health in and self-care with as it relates to people of color so important in the travel community?

Sometimes travel is used as an avoidance mechanism, people avoid the stress in their own lives by living for their next vacation. This isn't healthy, and frequent travelers should make sure they have identified why they are traveling.

Although we travel often for our mental health, the topic is not emphasized due to shame and stigma. How can we normalize this conversation among the travel communities of color?

Normalizing this conversation requires more honesty from everyone.

Roshida Dowe

WEBSITE

www.shidasontheloose.com

EMAIL

roshida@shidasontheloose.com

INSTAGRAM HANDLE

@ShidaD

FACEBOOK PAGE

facebook.com/shidasontheloose

Travel Jokes

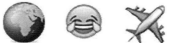

CHAPTER 52

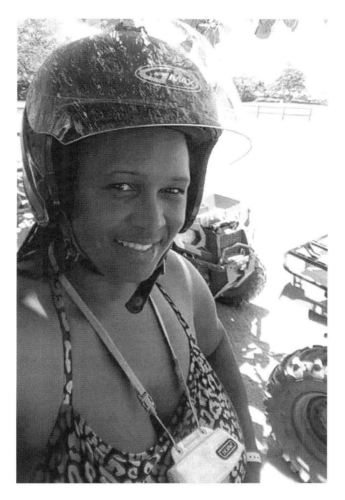

Javonne Sanders

Mobile Salad Bar

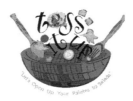

Travel Quote or Travel Mantra you live by
Toss It Up, Toss Out the Fear and Book it.

Travel Influencer/ Brand Summary

> Toss it Up Salad Bar is a mobile salad bar providing mouthwatering healthy nutritious salads to the community of Los Angeles which will Toss Up the health epidemics that are affecting the youth, middle and elderly citizens. I want to show people in my community a different way of life through eating healthy and traveling the world

How has Traveling helped you maintain your mental health as it relates to self-care?

> Traveling has helped me while doing business by escaping from the stressful and busy everyday living.

What is your most therapeutic travel destination for stress relief and self-care?

> I like to visit warm tropical places where I can have fun and enjoy the excursions and take time to get a nice full massage afterward.

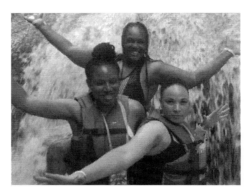

Whats is the most important items you have in your carryon and why?

> I would say the most important thing for me would be my toiletries and a change of clothes. Just in case I do have a layover, I can change into a clean pair of underwear.

Favorite Calming Beverage or Food to consume while traveling and why?

> I really do not have a calming beverage or food. I enjoy

Favorite Calming Music or Audio to listen to while traveling?

> I do not have a playlist while traveling. When I am in the country that I visiting, I listen to their station so I can get the experience of the people who reside there.

Favorite Keepsake that keeps you calm or grounded while traveling?

> I say a prayer for safety and speak that I will arrive at my destination in a timely matter.

Javonne Sanders

What is your most hilarious travel memory?

> There is soo many I can't narrow it down but I was probably with my cousin

What is your most memorable or touching travel experience?

> The most memorable experience would be traveling with my cousin. It's touching for me because I met my cousin a couple of years ago on Facebook and I never thought that I would ever experience that with a family member.

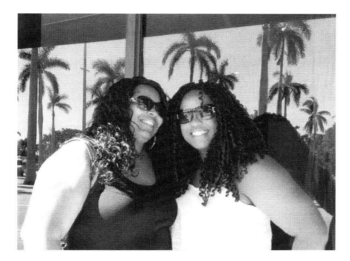

What is the worst travel experience you ever had?

> I try to look at the glass half full than empty. I haven't experienced anything regards to travel as long as I can arrive back home safely... I am Ok.

Favorite Travel Hack?

> Uber

What is your travel Ritual for keeping calm and maintaining your inner zen?

> My travel ritual for keeping calm and maintaining my inner zen would be to realize that there are things we can not control.

Best Travel Tip Advice

> Go with a positive attitude and realize that things just happen

Why is addressing mental health in and self-care with as it relates to people of color so important in the travel community?

> Addressing mental health and self-care is so important because we are all facing something in our everyday lives. Since there is a vast amount of people of color who do travel and might know others who are facing difficulties and need to relax and unwind.

Although we travel often for our mental health, the topic is not emphasized due to shame and stigma. How can we normalize this conversation among the travel communities of color?

> This could be normalized by giving tips on how to travel economically and how to plan and the importance of traveling. Many of color might feel like the planning process is harder than what it is and why we all need to get away from the hustle and bustle of the everyday lifestyle.

WEBSITE

www.tossitupinc.com

EMAIL

jsanders821@ymail.com

INSTAGRAM HANDLE

Tossitupsalad

Travel Jokes

Delta flights be like:
We are now taking
- Pre Boarding
- Military and Parents with small children
- Diamond & First Class
- Comfort+
- Sky Priority
- Business Class
- Xbox Gold Live Members
- Tea Party Members
- Taylor Swift Fans
- Disney + paid subscribers
- BlackBerry Curve users
- Sacramento Kings Fans
- Four Loko drinkers
- Everest College Graduates
- MAIN CABIN 1

CHAPTER 53

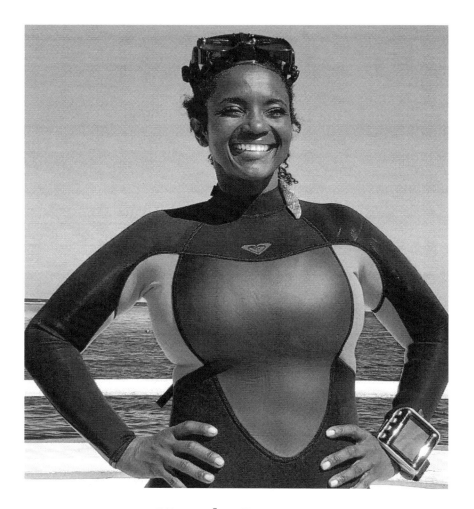

Hooda Brown

Black Girls Scuba too

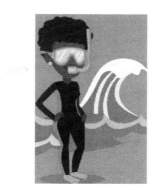

Black Girls Scuba 2

Travel Quote or Travel Mantra you live by

I want to See It, Feel It, Smell It, Hear It and Taste all that this world and this life has to offer for myself.

Travel Influencer/ Brand Summary

My primary purpose in sharing my travel experiences is to draw parallels between the experiences I've had in life. Secondly to inspire young black girls and women around the world to learn how to scuba dive and live their wildest dreams. There are universal themes that can be applied by any and everyone to LIVE out the time we are given.

How has Traveling helped you maintain your mental health as it relates to self-care?

As a divorcee of nearly 14 years now when I think back to my early quick trips away just to go aimlessly walk the streets of NYC I began to realize how important it was to disconnect and learn new things. Business owner, mother of 2 had me in a constant state of fatigue, anxious and overwhelmed with the day to day nonstop obligations to the needs of others. Emotional spent most days was my state of being at the time. Solo travel allowed me enough time to unplug and connect to myself in order to have something to give.

What is your most therapeutic travel destination for stress relief and self-care?

The Ocean. There is nothing manmade in the ocean there are no triangles, there are no squares, there are no rectangles. Everything has texture, color, depth and most importantly it's All ALIVE! Scuba diving provides these transient blocks of time where I am floating in slow motion yet keenly aware of my breaths, my depth and my Oxygen levels all the while visually taking in things that only 2% of the world's population will ever get to see up close. There are amazing things that you get an opportunity to SEE in the SEA.

Whats is the most important items you have in your carryon and why?

My buoyancy control device (BCD), dive computer and my regulator are the most important items in my carry on. The scuba equipment is not cheap so I don't want it damaged lost or stolen so it goes on the plane with me.

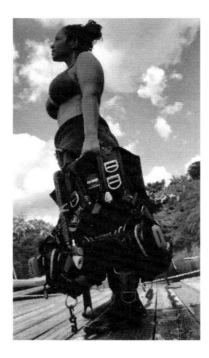

Favorite Calming Beverage or Food to consume while traveling and why?

Two parts Hydrogen and One part Oxygen (H2O) is my favorite beverage when I'm traveling because my travel tends to lean more towards adventure travel.

Favorite Calming Music or Audio to listen to while traveling?

My favorite music to listen to when I travel is world beat music like Bossanova. Instrumentals are my preference in that I would rather not process words just hear pleasants sounds.

Favorite Keepsake that keeps you calm or grounded while traveling?

I am not a tricket person.

What is your most hilarious travel memory?

Standing at the Pyramids of Giza near the Sphinx and slowly becoming "the attraction". I Was standing with my selfie stick taking tourist pictures with the Sphinx and I started to notice that this group of young Egyptian girls were staring at me with these big smiles all giggling. After about 10 mins one came over and asked for a selfie with me and that was like turning on the flood gates. For the next 45 minutes, I was taking selfies with them and just about every Egyptian that passed by. They kept making note of how beautiful I was and how beautiful my skin was. It was hilarious to me to be standing next to a W midtown under of The World and folks wanted to take photos with me... go figure!🤳♀️🤣

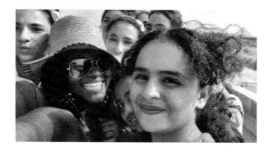

What is your most memorable or touching travel experience?

I am a master scuba diver and for the last 10 years, I have been traveling and diving alone just with random people on boats. Well this year I joined the national association of black scuba divers in June and they were getting ready for a trip in November to dive The Red Sea in Sharm El Shiek, Eygpt. The red sea was 1# on my bucket list so finally dive the Red Sea with 120 other people that look like me was an amazing experience.

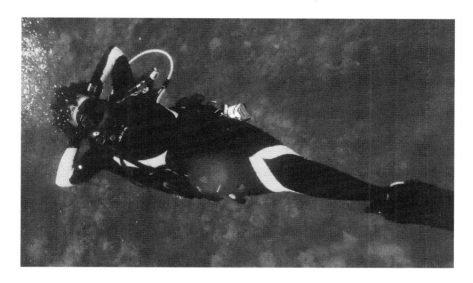

What is the worst travel experience you ever had?

I was traveling back from Niseko Japan snowboarding and my daughter had a performance that she was really nervous about and there was a storm delay and missed connections and no flights out of Tokyo so I spent the night in Tokyo and missed my baby's stage debut.

Favorite Travel Hack?

Momondo always saves me money on flights

What is your travel Ritual for keeping calm and maintaining your inner zen?

My travel ritual is to begin every trip with great expectations and excitement because I feel like I draw amazing experience to me with that energy. I drink a lot of water and eat mostly fish and I've yet to have an upset stomach.

Best Travel Tip Advice?

Simply Go. Tomorrow is not promised to prioritize doing some of the things you want to do in this life. Make down payments of you need to but GO!

Why is addressing mental health in and self-care with as it relates to people of color so important in the travel community?

The trauma and stress of being black in America is a weighted experience as microaggressions are almost non stop on a daily basis. I feel its incredibly important that we take time to create our own experiences abroad and do something different than the mind-numbing sameness of working.

Although we travel often for our mental health, the topic is not emphasized due to shame and stigma. How can we normalize this conversation among the travel communities of color?

Honesty. If people would be more honest with themselves and recognize when you need a moment for you then we are better prepared to share and ask for help when life is simply too much

Travel Jokes

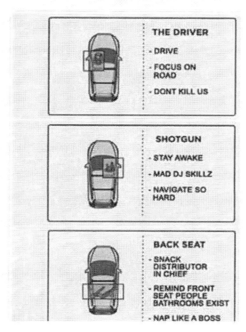

We have now landed in Optimal Mental health Wellness. Thanks for flying Let's Get Mental Airlines. We hope you enjoyed your flight.

THE END

The end of suffering in silence, stigma and shame

Mental Health Awareness Observances & Resources and Apps

Mental health Awareness Month – May

Minority Mental Health Awareness Month – July

Mental Health Awareness Week -First full week of Oct

World Suicide Prevention Day Sept 10th

National Suicide Prevention week- 2nd week of Sept

Mental Health Awareness Apparel & Office Swag

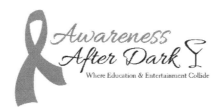

https://awarenessafterdarkapparel.com/

Apps

Ayana Therapy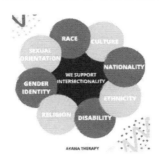

Safe Place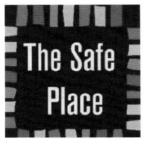

Podcast

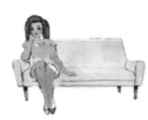 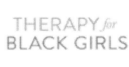 
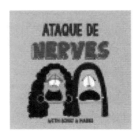 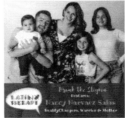 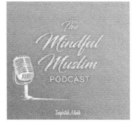
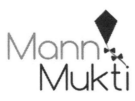 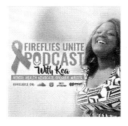 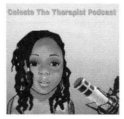

Mental Health Awareness Observances & Resources and Apps

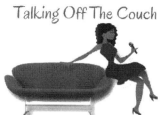
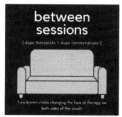
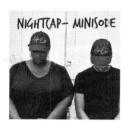
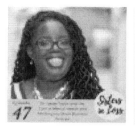
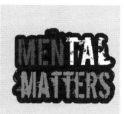

Conferences

Los Angeles County Department of Mental Health Bi-Annual African American Mental Health Conference

Can We Talk Conference and Benefit Dinner

Black Mental Health Symposium

Organizations

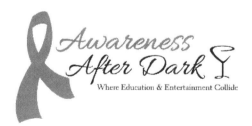

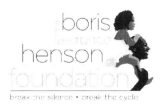

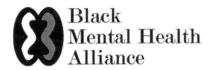

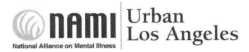

Documentaries

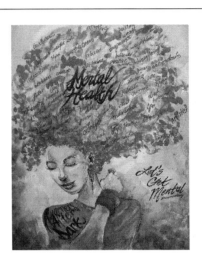
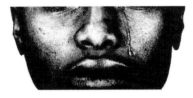

International Hotlines

USA

1-800-273-8255
Suicide Prevention Lifeline

UK

08457 90 90 90
Samartians

0800 068 4141
HopeLine UK

EUROPE

Emergency Numbers
European Emergency Number: 112

France (English Speaking)

0033 145 39 4000
Suicide Ecoute

01 46 21 46 46
SOS Help

Germany

Telefonseelsorge Deutschland (National)

German speaking: 0800 -111 0 222
English speaking: 030-44 01 06 07
Crisis support line 6pm to 12am daily

Italy

800 86 00 22
Samaritans

SOUTH AFRICA

0861 322 322
Lifeline Southern Africa

Made in the USA
Monee, IL
29 October 2020

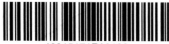